What Every Medical Writer Needs to Know

Robert B. Taylor

What Every Medical Writer Needs to Know

Questions and Answers for the Serious Medical Author

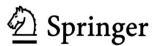 Springer

Robert B. Taylor, MD
Professor
Department of Family and Community Medicine
Eastern Virginia Medical School
Norfolk, VA, USA

Professor Emeritus
Department of Family Medicine
Oregon Health & Science University
School of Medicine
Portland, OR, USA

ISBN 978-3-319-20263-1   ISBN 978-3-319-20264-8   (eBook)
DOI 10.1007/978-3-319-20264-8

Library of Congress Control Number: 2015945099

Springer Cham Heidelberg New York Dordrecht London

Printed on acid-free paper

Springer International Publishing AG Switzerland is part of Springer Science+Business Media
(www.springer.com)

Medicine and writing go well together, they shed light on each other and both do better by going hand in hand. A doctor possessed of the writer's art will be the better consoler to anyone rolling in agony; conversely, a writer who understands the life of the body, its powers and its pains, its fluids and functions, its blessings and banes, has a great advantage over him who knows nothing of such things.

—German writer Thomas Mann,
author of *The Magic Mountain*

I think all writing is a disease. You can't stop it.

—American physician and poet
William Carlos Williams

For Frankie, Masha, Jack, and Annie

Preface

Anyone can learn to dance. Each of us can grow roses. And any medical or journalism professional—with years of education that included at least a few writing assignments—can be a medical writer. The hard part is to "Dance with the Stars," grow roses that are the envy of your neighbors, or write outstanding medical articles, books, and technical reports.

This book is intended to increase your understanding of the art of medical writing. It is not a "how-to" book about medical writing; I already write one of those, titled *Medical Writing: A Guide for Clinicians, Educators, and Researchers, 2nd edition* [1]. This book is different in that it is *about* medical writing—about what we do, why and how we do it, the goals we seek, the perils we face, and what we can learn from others who have walked the trail before us.

One of the themes of this book is that we medical writers can learn a lot from past and current authors whose works are, for some reason, recognized as both noteworthy in content and skillfully crafted. Yes, medical writing is "different," partly because our profession is considered enigmatic by the uninitiated, and perhaps because the vocabulary we use is so different from the words most people speak each day. At its core, medical writing is thinking through a topic, perhaps performing a research study, and, in the past, putting words on paper and today on a computer screen.

The fundamentals of writing transcend the various backgrounds of those who aspire to author works for others to read. Medical writing is not so special that we cannot learn from some of the "great" authors such as Robert Frost, Gertrude Stein, and Marcel Proust, as well as familiar medical writers such as Sir William Osler, Elizabeth Kübler-Ross, and Abraham Verghese.

Who needs this book? The answer is anyone who is serious about medical writing. It is for anyone who should know about rookie mistakes, medical authorisms, publication bias, the Dizzy Awards, and the Gunning Fog Index, how being a medical writer is like being a surgeon, the basics of technical medical writing, the facts about predatory publishers, and new pitfalls writers and academicians face in copyright infringement. The potential reader is anyone who wants to know what Doctor W. Somerset Maugham told of the three basic rules of good writing, how Doctor

Anton Chekhov described his dual lives in medicine and literature, and the story behind the curious writings of Doctor Egerton Yorrick Davis. What medical writer helped finance his medical school education by selling blood and publishing poems in popular magazines such as *Saturday Evening Post* and *Harper's Bazaar*? [It was Lewis Thomas, who went on to become dean of not one, but two medical schools.] What medical researcher wrote a poem to commemorate a breakthrough discovery he had just made? [Sir Ronald Ross wrote his poem in 1897 after observing the malarial parasite growing in a mosquito.] Knowing these facts and tales can only make you a more knowledgeable medical author.

The paragraph above describes a diverse group of people and stories. In fact, there is no prototypical medical writer. Instead, medical writers — and the audience for this book — include researchers preparing their data for publication, clinicians with an observation to report, professional medical writers preparing regulatory or educational documents, health professionals with the itch to pen a book of stories from practice or medicine-themed fiction, and more. And because medical writers often lead schizophrenic lives — think of William Carlos Williams writing poetry such as *So Much Depends* while waiting to deliver a baby — their stories are often colorful.

I hope that this book will enrich your life as a medical writer, and that you find a few stories in the pages to come that make you feel a little more connected with the community of medical writers everywhere, both in the past and today. Simply stated, I hope you enjoy the book.

Virginia Beach, VA, USA   Robert B. Taylor

Reference

1. Taylor RB. Medical writing: a guide for clinicians, educators, and researchers, Ed 2. New York: Springer; 2011.

Contents

List of Figures

Chapter 1
About Medical Writing and Writers

Catherine DeAngelis, Editor in Chief of the *Journal of the American Medical Association* (JAMA), has stated, "I never cease to be amazed by the general inability of physicians, other health professionals, and scientists to communicate through the written word" [1]. Having a pile of data is not enough, knowing the IMRaD model (Introduction, Methods, Results, and Discussion) is just a start, and the *AMA Manual of Style* can only offer guidelines for writing for a specific type of medical publication. In the end, success in medical writing calls for both basic composition skills and knowledge of the history and landscape of the enterprise. This first chapter provides a look into the world of medical writing, starting with our reaching agreement on terms I will use in the book, and then examining characteristics of excellent medical writing and the traits of those who have successfully mastered the skills to create these works.

What Is Medical Writing and What Is Special About It?

Medical writing is written communication that addresses some health-related topic that is intended to be read by anyone interested in medicine, science, or the process of health care delivery. Thus medical writing's subject matter and audience are quite diverse. Here are some examples of influential medical writing over the past few centuries.

Country doctor Edward Jenner's observation on cowpox and his subsequent publication in 1798 of *An Inquiry Into the Causes and Effects of the Variolae Vaccinae* changed a world that had lived in fear of smallpox [2] (see Fig. 1.1).

In 1860, following his observations and an unplanned controlled experiment that supported his thesis, Ignaz Semmelweis published his monograph, *The Etiology, the Concept, and the Prophylaxis of Childbed Fever* [4]. The book detailed how pregnant women delivered by medical students coming directly from performing autopsies to deliver babies had a much higher rate of puerperal infection than those

© Springer International Publishing Switzerland 2015
R.B. Taylor, *What Every Medical Writer Needs to Know*,
DOI 10.1007/978-3-319-20264-8_1

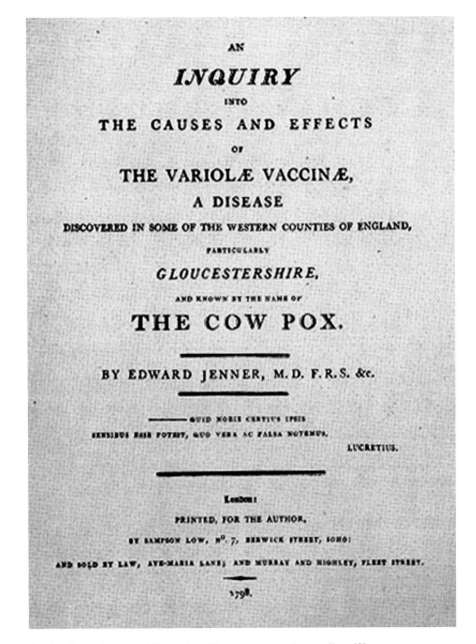

Fig. 1.1 Report by Edward Jenner describing a vaccine against smallpox [3]

delivered by midwives who had no autopsy duties. All this changed when Semmelweis instituted hand washing by the medical students, and the results are described in his 500-page treatise.

Fielding Garrison, in 1913, singlehandedly penned *An Introduction to History of Medicine,* a painstakingly researched and richly illustrated epic work, even though the subject was not "clinical" [5]. The book, much more than an introduction, continued through its fourth edition (1929).

In 1936, Wingate M. Johnson wrote *The True Physician: The Modern "Doctor of the Old School,"* extolling the traditional values of medicine [6]. The first report to clearly link *Helicobacter pylori (H. pylori)* to peptic ulcer disease, authored by Australian physicians Barry Marshall, appeared in 1985 [7]. Then in 2008, Richard Smith, long-time editor of the British Medical Journal, wrote an article "The Trouble With Medical Journals," published in the *Medico-Legal Journal* [8].

On April 30, 2014, the *Wall Street Journal* published a letter from Ardis Dee Hoven, MD, President of the American Medical Association, titled "New Models of Health-Care Delivery," discussing workings of the US Center for Medicare and Medicaid Innovation and prospects for strengthening the US health care system in general [9]. Is this medical writing only because a physician penned it? No, it would also qualify as medical writing if the author were a journalist or professional medical writer.

And then there is the intriguing chapter in the history of brain surgery, *The Tale of the Dueling Neurosurgeons,* by writer Sam Kean [10]. The "dueling neurosurgeons" are Ambroise Paré and Andreas Vesalius; the author is neither a physician nor a surgeon, but I consider his work to be a type of medical writing.

In fact, all of the above are examples of medical writing. The chief common denominator is not that the authors are all health professionals, but that the *topics* are all health related in some way. The various subjects medical writers write about are important not only for those involved in patient care and health care policy, but also for everyone. Every person has a stake in new treatments, such as the antibiotic therapy of peptic ulcer disease that followed discovery that there is a causative relationship between *H. pylori* and peptic ulcer disease. Every clinician should know the "trouble with medical journals" described by Richard Smith, and which I will discuss in more detail in Chap. 5. All Americans are affected by what's happening in health care delivery, as told by Ardis Dee Hoven. And all who write about these topics are medical writers.

Who Is a Medical Writer?

Anyone who writes about medical science, education, history, or practice is a medical writer. That includes researchers describing the results of laboratory and clinical trials, educators telling about how they teach and reporting the outcomes of their efforts, clinicians who write to describe what they have discovered in practice, and every health professional who pens a novel with a medical theme. But that is not all.

Many medical writers—sometimes called medical communicators—are employed by industry, writing informational reports describing drugs and devices, preparing written materials related to clinical trials submitted to the US Food and

Drug Administration (FDA), or creating other documents such as investigator brochures and technical reports. Most persons making a living as medical writers, and not as clinicians, have MSc, PhD, or similar degrees. Some have no advanced degrees and have learned on the job, but these persons are the exceptions [11].

Who Are Some of the Great Medical Writers of History?

The pages of history tell of remarkable medical writers, whom we remember for the new ideas they introduced, the timelessness of the thoughts they expressed, and their extraordinary productivity. Here are just a few of them.

- **Hippocrates**. Hippocrates of Kos (c. 460–c. 370 BCE), who held that afflictions were not caused by the wrath of angry gods but by natural causes, described many diseases and abnormalities, such as what we now call "Hippocratic fingers." He is credited with some 70 medical writings, although it is not clear whether he or his acolytes wrote the actual documents [12] (see Fig. 1.2).

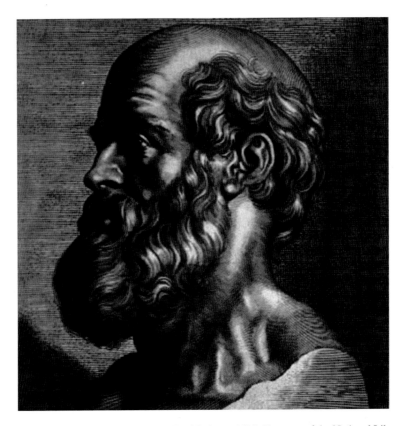

Fig. 1.2 Hippocrates, engraving by Peter Paul Rubens, 1638. Courtesy of the National Library of Medicine [13]

- **Galen**. The most prolific medical writer of Roman times was Greek physician Galen of Pergamon (129–c. 200), who penned more than 300 works of various types, comprising approximately 8000 pages. He wrote on anatomy, circulation of blood, and the nervous system [14]. He wrote this all by hand and, whether his theories were correct or not, because of the intellectual famine of the mediaeval times that followed, they prevailed for a thousand years.
- **Avicenna and Maimonides**. As the seat of learning moved to the Middle East during the Dark Ages in Europe, Avicenna (980–1037) in Persia wrote more than 400 works, notably the *Canon of Medicine*, which Sir William Osler once called "the most famous medical textbook ever written" [15]. More than a century later, physician and Rabbi Moses ben Maimon, aka Maimonides (1138–1204) and his family fled religious persecution in Spain and settled eventually in Egypt, where he wrote ten medical works on topics such as poisons, asthma, fits, hemorrhoids, and the aphorisms of Hippocrates [16].
- **Thomas Sydenham**. Sometimes called the "English Hippocrates" and the "father of English medicine," Thomas Sydenham (1624–1689) published *Observations on Medicine* in 1676 (see Fig. 1.3). He wrote on a wide variety of subjects: fevers, epidemics, venereal diseases, dropsy (edema), arthritis, pulmonary consumption (tuberculosis), gout, and smallpox. He named "scarlet fever" as a disease, differentiating it from measles [18].
- **Sir William Osler**. As we approach more recent medical writing, we come to Sir William Osler, the Canadian-born physician who played a leading role in founding Johns Hopkins Hospital in Baltimore. He has been called the

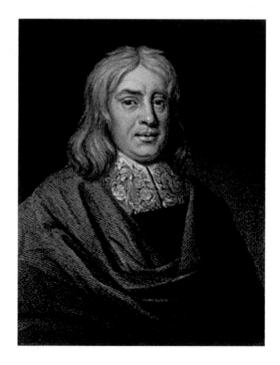

Fig. 1.3 Thomas Sydenham, seventieth-century English physician [17]

"father of modern medicine." In the pantheon of famous medical writers, Osler is noteworthy as the sole author of the reference book *The Principles and Practice of Medicine,* first published in 1892, and continuing in print, in various editions, for more than 40 years [19]. In addition to being a writer, Osler was an educator, aphorist, and prankster.

Today, some modern medical writers have become household names, at least in my household: William Carlos Williams, Elizabeth Kübler-Ross, Richard Selzer, Jerome Groopman, Atul Gawande, Abraham Verghese, and others. I will return to some of these inspirational medical writers, including Osler, later in the book.

How Has the Process of Writing Changed Over the Years?

How we write has undergone profound changes over the millennia. Some of the first writing, dating to Mesopotamia some five millennia ago, is described as "cuneiform," from the Latin word *cuneus,* meaning wedge. The writing instrument was a wedge-shaped stylus used to make impressions on clay, stone, or wax. Although chiefly used for business—such as recording sales of goats or barley—some medical texts recorded on tablets have been preserved [20].

Subsequent major changes in writing and publication occurred with the development of papyrus as a writing material. This advance occurred in early Egypt, and allowed the use of ink. A medical writer who described various ailments of his time was the Egyptian physician Imhotep, who lived in around the twenty-seventh century BCE. What remains today, probably copied from earlier documents, is called the Edwin Smith papyrus, commemorating the explorer who found the document (see Fig. 1.4).

Later, in Europe, papyrus as a writing material was replaced by longer lasting parchment and, subsequently, paper, setting the stage for the introduction of moveable-type mechanical printing technology—aka the printing press—by Johannes Gutenberg in 1450.

A more recent major advance was the introduction of the typewriter in the 1860s, and the art of handwriting began to fade. All but thank-you notes and family letters came to be typed. The old-fashioned typewriter, with long, swinging arms that tended to jam and ink ribbons that needed frequent replacement, gave way to the text-editing typewriter, and then word processors and personal computers. Many of us have lived through this transition, grateful, but often also challenged, by each new enhancement to our productivity.

The Internet has been the game changer for all types of communication, including writing. One author estimates that, worldwide, there are ten billion devices—computers, smartphones, tablets, and more—connected via the Internet [22]. I edit a major—1200+ pages—reference book in family medicine, *Family Medicine: Principles and Practice,* initially published in 1976. The manuscript for the first edition, almost 3000 pages, filled two large, heavy cardboard boxes. Because only one copy existed, I delivered the original manuscript to the publisher by hand, to

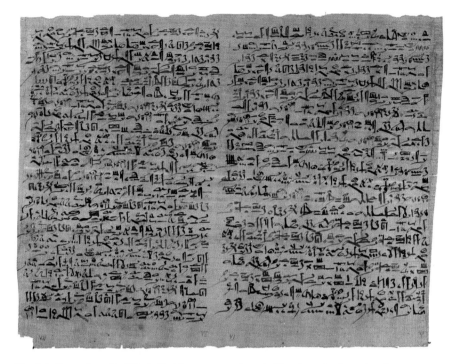

Fig. 1.4 Pages from the Edwin Smith papyrus, written in hieratic script in ancient Egypt around 1600 BCE [21]

avoid risking loss in the mail. Today, manuscripts are prepared on computer and submitted electronically—no paper at all.

Today my teenage grandchildren struggle to write a letter in cursive, although they can text like champions. In a generation, will my great-grandchildren be able to read handwriting at all?

The Internet has also changed how medical writing is published. We, an expanded editorial team, are currently preparing the 7th edition of the *Family Medicine* book. It is being assembled initially for online publication. Then, when the online version is complete and on the "platform," a traditional paper book will be released.

We have come a long way since the days of the clay tablet and wedge-shaped stylus.

What Changes Have We Seen Over the Past Few Decades in the Nature and Process of Medical Writing?

During my professional lifetime, I have witnessed a number of changes in medical writing and publication. These trends are important because they indicate topics of greater or lesser interest to readers; they also suggest opportunities and challenges for aspiring authors. Here is what I have noticed:

A Robust Proliferation in the Number of Medical and Scientific Journals

The oldest scientific journal in continuing publication is *The Philosophical Transactions of the Royal Society,* abbreviated Phil. Trans., and first published in London on March 6, 1665. Charles Darwin and Isaac Newton were among the writers who contributed to this journal [23] (see Fig. 1.5).

Today there are an estimated 25–40,000 scientific journals, of which 96 % are published online, and some 10 % are open access [25]. In addition to JAMA, *New England Journal of Medicine* (NEJM), and the *British Medical Journal* (BMJ), there are, among the less widely read journals, *The Journal of Nicotine and Tobacco Research, The International Journal of Health Services, Neuropsychopharmacology, Positivity, Retina, Pain,* and *Gut.*

Fewer Case Reports and New Diseases Described

In the past many journals published case reports regularly, and this provided the neophyte medical writer with an opportunity to achieve publication. In 2012, Sivasubramanian et al. described a meniscal cyst of the knee joint misdiagnosed as a Baker cyst [26]. Few such case reports find their way into print today.

Also seldom encountered is the epiphanic description of a new disease. There are a few. Recently we have seen reports of MERS, aka the Middle East respiratory syndrome. No single person's name is attached to these reports, and the occasional new disease reported is instead identified by an acronym: MERS, MRSA (methicillin-resistant *Staphylococcus aureus*), or SARS (severe acute respiratory syndrome). The sort of disease description that might once have earned one an eponymous disease name—Hashimoto thyroiditis or Sydenham chorea—is becoming less common in medical writing today.

Multiple Authors

The top journals now compete to publish the major, multi-institutional studies, and this means that many investigators are involved. As an example, a 2014 report by Asfar et al. in the *New England Journal of Medicine* on mortality rates associated with different blood pressure targets in patients with septic shock listed 31 authors, with additional investigators "listed in the Supplementary Appendix, available at NEJM.org" [27].

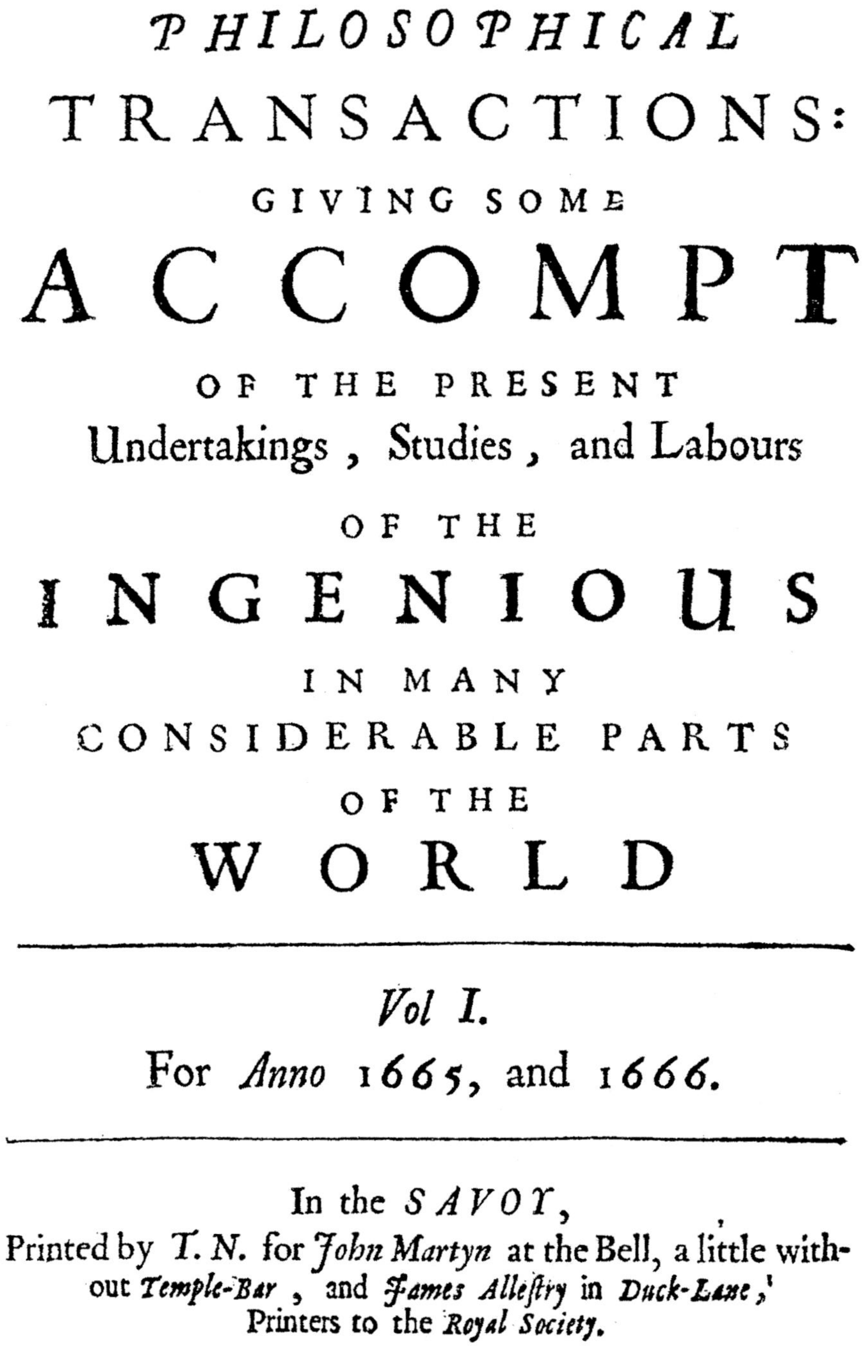

P HILOSOPHICAL

TRANSACTIONS:

GIVING SOME

ACCOMPT

OF THE PRESENT

Undertakings , Studies , and Labours

OF THE

INGENIOUS

IN MANY

CONSIDERABLE PARTS

OF THE

WORLD

Vol I.

For *Anno* 1665, and 1666.

In the *SAVOY*,

Printed by *T. N.* for *John Martyn* at the Bell, a little without *Temple-Bar* , and *James Allestry* in *Duck-Lane*,
Printers to the *Royal Society.*

Fig. 1.5 Philosophical Transactions of the Royal Society, Volume I, 1665 and 1666 [24]

More Complex Reports

Today's scientific journals strive for scholarly works that will withstand statistical scrutiny, both during peer review and after publication. Hence the articles, and especially the abstracts, are best described as dense. Clarity yields to data specificity. Here are the first two sentences in the Results section of the Asfar et al. blood pressure target/septic shock article mentioned above, hardly an example of eloquent prose [27]:

> At 28 days, there was no significant between-group difference in mortality, with deaths reported in 142 of 388 patients in the high-target group (36.6 %) and 132 of 388 patients in the low-target group (34.0 %) (hazard ratio in the high-target group, 1.07; 95 % confidence interval [CI], 0.84–1.38; $P=0.57$). There was also no significant difference in mortality at 90 days, with 170 deaths (43.8 %) and 164 deaths (43.3 %), respectively (hazard ratio, 1.04; 95 % CI, 0.83–1.30; $P=0.74$).

The selection of the Asfar et al. article to use as an example was not the result of a diligent search for an egregious example of hyper-authorism and abstract complexity. In fact, this example is typical of reports of major studies published today.

More Systematic Reviews, Meta-Analyses, and Now Umbrella Reviews

The systematic review is really a literature review looking at previously published reports on a specific topic. A meta-analysis applies statistical analysis to data from previous studies: "research about research." Thus a meta-analysis arises from a systemic review, but a systemic review does not necessarily prompt a meta-analysis of findings.

Two factors have fueled the rise of published systematic reviews and meta-analyses. The first is the current focus on evidence-based medicine, the quest to make clinical decisions based on the latest research findings—rather than tradition, experience, or expert opinion. The second impetus has been the success of the Cochrane Collaboration, founded in 1993 and named for Scottish physician and author Archie Cochrane, which most primary care physicians consider a highly reliable source of systematic reviews and evidence-based clinical information. The Cochrane Collaboration is described on their website as follows [28]:

> Cochrane is a global independent network of health practitioners, researchers, patient advocates and others, responding to the challenge of making the vast amounts of evidence generated through research useful for informing decisions about health. We are a not-for-profit organization with collaborators from over 120 countries working together to produce credible, accessible health information that is free from commercial sponsorship and other conflicts of interest.

The many systematic reviews now in print and online have spawned the "umbrella review," an analysis of previously published systematic reviews and meta-analyses.

Here is an example: In the *British Medical Journal*, Theodoratou et al. published an umbrella review of existing reports regarding vitamin D and various health outcomes [29]. All of this seems an enticing opportunity to conduct research and publish scholarly papers without entering an actual laboratory or sacrificing a single white rat.

Fewer Book Reviews

Book review columns were once a feature of most medical journals. Each medical book author or editor waited anxiously to learn what some peer selected to review the book would have to say. Did the reviewer like the book, perhaps gently suggesting some change to improve the next edition? Or was the review unfavorable, indicating, of course, that the reviewer was an illiterate troglodyte who apparently did not read the book at all?

The first change came when book review sections added reviews of media and web offerings. Then journal publishers gave up altogether, and today very few medical journals publish book reviews. As a medical writer, I, of course, believe this to be a great loss to the medical literature.

The Near-Total Demise of "Throw-Away" Medical Journals

A few decades ago, practicing physicians could expect the mail to bring one of the "throw-away" journals almost daily. Among their ranks were *The Female Patient, Physician's Management, Drug Therapy, Resident and Staff Physician,* and *Hippocrates.* The "throw-away" journals were entirely supported by advertising revenue, published only review articles (of varying quality), were rarely cited in the medical literature, and were generally not indexed in PubMed. These publications sound somewhat dubious, until you realize that, with their voracious appetite for clinical articles, they provided many neophyte physician writers with an opportunity to see their work in print.

Public Access to Many Published Works

On PubMed I can find the abstract to almost any medical article published in the last decade or so. I simply type the lead author name and article title into the "search" field. The same process works in Google Scholar. In many instances, however, my attempt to view the entire article leads me to a field asking me for a one-time fee for viewing the article, or inviting me to subscribe to the journal in which the article is published.

But things are changing. More and more medical articles, such as the "Baker cyst" article mentioned above, are published in open-access journals—meaning free, unrestricted access, and use. For example PLOS (Public Library of Science) publishes a suite of open-access journals covering subjects such as medicine, genetics, and neglected tropical diseases. One source estimates that 20 % of science articles are available free of charge [25].

Even many books, often works of historic interest, are available freely online. For example, *The Informed Writer: Using Sources in the Discipline*, by Charles Bazerman, is available in an open-access edition [30].

More Professional Medical Writers

In the past, being a medical writer generally meant being a physician who wrote. Today there are more professional medical writers without "medical" degrees than ever before, filling vital roles in research and industry. In fact, a randomly selected report of a major clinical trial published recently may, in fact, not have been composed by the researchers who conducted the study, but by a professional medical writer presenting the research findings using specialized skills in written communication.

Is There a Characteristic Personality Type That Describes Writers?

There is writing, and then there is good writing. There is evidence that perhaps some people have natural gifts that allow them to be more successful at writing than others [31]. But all of us have the ability to write; it is just easier when we recognize how our traits influence our writing behavior.

One of the most studied methods of describing personality types is the Myers-Briggs Type Indicator (MBTI). At its core, the MBTI employs dichotomous responses in four categories to describe how one gets one's energy (introvert, I, vs. extravert, E), sees the world (intuitive, N, vs. sensing, S), makes decisions about what is seen (thinking, T, vs. feeling, F), and lives his or her life (judging, J, or perceiving, P).

Youngblood describes a survey of writers, finding that they were somewhat different than the general population [31]. In Youngblood's study, the most common MBTI type was the INTJ, representing 24.9 % of all writers responding, compared with 2 % in the general population. In MBTI parlance, the INTJ is the "mastermind"—introverted, preferring abstract material and sensing possibilities, thinking in an objective manner, and being uncomfortable until a decision is made. What does this show about the strengths of this personality type as a writer? INTJs tend to start working on a project early and will deliver it on time; make an outline after planning extensively in their heads; have a clear, organized style; and excel at writing about theories and ideas. Their drawbacks are that their progress can be "blocked" by too much advice from others or by the search for an original angle, and their desire for closure may prevent them from revising their work sufficiently. I am an INTJ, and you will see this style reflected in my writing.

In the survey, the next most common MBTI type was INFJ (the "counselor"), representing 23.9 % of writers versus 1.5 % of the general population. INFJs differ from INTJs in that they are more likely to make writing decisions based empathically on feelings. Like the INTJs, they tend to plan their writing project before starting to write and they require time alone to develop their ideas. However, they may spend countless hours searching for the perfect words and revising the document because they are so personally connected to their writing. Youngblood speculates that the single difference between the two writer groups—thinkers vs. feelers—might reflect gender differences.

Note that there are 16 MBTI personality types, and yet almost half of all writers are found in two of these types. Yes, there seems to be a "writer's personality."

What Are the Strengths of and Challenges for Different Personality Types When It Comes to Medical Writing?

Individuals in each MBTI type have their "preferred" approach to medical writing—and to living life [32, 33].

- *Extraverts* tend to write best when ideas or material comes from discussing the topics with someone else and when writing quickly with little or no planning. They can clarify and polish their written draft later. It is important for an extravert to take frequent breaks when writing. Extraverts can be helped by making an oral presentation on their topic before trying to write. Outlines might be written after a first draft is produced. A pitfall for extraverts is trying to include too much in a writing project and not developing their thesis fully.
- *Intraverts*, as described above, want their ideas clear before writing, but they may plan excessively and never get anything on paper.
- *Sensors* do best when given specific, crystal-clear instructions and a prescribed format to follow. They can be confused by vague directions and overwhelmed by too much material. They are most effective writing about practical reality-based topics.
- *Intuitives* like to write briskly and their ideas flow one to another. They can get diverted by making a topic more complex than it needs to be.
- *Thinkers* need to organize their thoughts and like outlines. They prefer to focus on concrete data. They need to believe that their writing will be evaluated fairly.
- *Feelers* prefer projects that have personal meaning, especially if it is from their own experience (such as "A Piece of Mind" in *JAMA* or "Pulse" on the Internet). They may fear rejection or that what they write will hurt someone's feelings.

- *Judgers* are attracted to focused topics. They set realistic goals, and keep their eyes on deadlines. They may, however, write before they have completed their research for the topic, jumping in to write when ideas are still undeveloped.
- *Perceivers* are drawn to broad topics and tend to engage in extensive research. They often get so involved in data accumulation that the original topic's boundaries and the project timeline become hazy [32, 33].

The MBTI is widely used today, and it is likely that you took the test in school or at work. If you are experiencing any difficulty with your writing, it might be helpful to revisit your results to see if your current writing problems are related to your fundamental personality type.

Do Some Writers Simply Feel Compelled to Get Words on Paper (or on Their Computer Screens)?

I think many do. Many writers rank sitting at their computers, creating something that had not previously existed, as among their favorite activities. I think of this as the "Zen of writing," or perhaps something like the "runner's high." Some writers feel an emptiness when not tapping keys with their fingers. According to American writer Wallace Stegner, "A day without work is a day lost, and some of the saddest people in the long history of mankind have been creators whose creativity wore out before they did" [34].

What Characterizes Good Writing of Any Type?

In general, the best writing has certain characteristics: First of all, the topic must have an *audience*. That is, someone must be willing to publish your work and that means that, one way or other, the company that publishes your work must make a little money. Somebody must pay for (and presumably read) the scientific journal, book, or electronic publication.

The second characteristic is *originality*. The best writing tells what has not been told before, or relates the twice-told tale with a new twist. How many books have been written about the death of President John F. Kennedy? Yet, in 2012 the television commentator Bill O'Reilly presented what some consider new insights in a bestselling book, *Killing Kennedy* [35].

The third characteristic of good writing is the use of *concrete examples* to illustrate assertions. State what you want to say and then back it up with an example. Note that under originality above, I described what I meant by the concept, and then I provided an example—the O'Reilly book—to illustrate my point. And I just used the previous sentence as an example of a "concrete example." Writing that lacks such examples soon becomes tedious, and the reader's attention wanders. The use of a case in point makes writing come alive.

Clarity is the fourth general characteristic of good writing. The best writer writes sparingly, and avoids long, complicated words and sentences that make the reader stop and reread to understand the message. If you can, write "short words" instead of "monosyllabic words." The latter might seem to be more erudite, but also can be just a little pedantic. In Chap. 4, I will tell about the *Gunning Fog Index* and how it can help you write for the educational level of your audience.

The fifth feature of good writing is *credibility*. Woe to the writer who misstates a known fact, such as crediting Marconi with inventing the telephone. Recently we saw the release of the American Psychiatric Association's *Diagnostic and Statistical Manual of Mental Disorders, 5th edition* (DSM-5), described in the publisher's marketing material as "the product of more than 10 years of effort by hundreds of international experts in all aspects of mental health" [36]. But the credibility of DSM-5 has been robustly challenged. Allen Frances, professor emeritus at Duke University, describes DSM-5 as "filled with glaring mistakes in wording and coding" and "remarkably amateurish." Citing the 4th edition of the book, Frances tells the problems that incorrect phrasing can cause [37]:

> Example—my greatest regret about DSM-IV was our inadvertent substitution of an "or" for an "and" in the criteria set for Paraphilia. This one stupid slip contributed to the unconstitutional preventive detention of thousands of sex offenders. I have no pity for criminals, but do have great concern when their constitutional rights are violated just because I made a dumb wording mistake.

Allen goes on to describe 18 errors in the DSM-5 document.

In Addition to the Above, What Are the Special Characteristics of Good Medical Writing?

Good medical writing reflects *evidence of planning*. Work published in the medical literature—whether it is the *Journal of the American Medical Association*, a specialty-specific reference book, or an industry summary of research regarding a new drug, the writing—will be read by some of the most knowledgeable and critical of all readers. Careful planning, and by this I mean thinking before writing, is especially important in the preparation of research reports, where the material must be presented in a prescribed format.

There must be evidence of a *thorough and timely literature search*. This must include one last journey through the current literature after acceptance of an article and just before publication.

The best medical writing reflects *careful word choice*. For example, "significance" describes the likelihood that a result could have occurred by chance, classically expressed as a p-value. When the good medical writer thinks something reported is important, but there is no statistical analysis offered, a better word would be "meaningful." Other words that have specific statistical and methodological connotations are "bias," "prevalence," "reliability," and "validity."

The *use of active voice*, even in research reports, characterizes skillful medical writing. An article in the *New England Journal of Medicine* on "Transcatheter Aortic-Valve Replacement with a Self-Expanding Prosthesis" offers a good example. In the abstract under Background we find, "We compared transcatheter aortic-valve replacement (TAVR)…," and later, under Methods, "We recruited patients with severe aortic stenosis…." Then in the body of the article, the use of first-person, active voice continues: "We hypothesized that a number of factors may have contributed…" [38].

Accuracy in what is said is vital in medical writing. A small error in a research report invites a flurry of letters to the editor, pointing out your transgression. A textbook with a dosage error can lead to episodes of drug toxicity. When it comes to books, we are reminded of the words of Mark Twain, "Be careful about reading health books. You may die of a misprint."

All medical authors should be *factual in summarizing conclusions of findings*. It also is generally appropriate to be succinct and unassuming. Adams et al. end their paper comparing their self-expanding prosthesis with traditional surgical aortic-valve replacement (TAVR) with this sentence, "The rate of death from any cause at 1 year was significantly reduced with TAVR performed with the self-expanding prosthesis" [38]. There is no call for the former surgical method to be abandoned, no speculation as to how many lives might be saved using TAVR, just a simple statement of fact, with use of the word "significantly" based on presentation of *p*-values described in the paper.

What Do You Like Most About Being a Medical Writer?

Every day and every project is different. I am a generalist physician and I relish variety in what I encounter in practice. In the office, never a day passes without seeing some new combination of disease problems or perhaps psychosocial issues.

My writing interests are also varied: Over a four-decade writing career, I have written or edited two books on medical writing, three on medical history and philosophy, four on diagnosis, and six editions of a major reference book in my specialty.

Much of my writing today is books like this one—topical and referenced—projects that help me learn new things. I seem to alternate between three areas: clinical diagnosis, medical history, and medical writing. Every day at the computer is an adventure, a journey to the far reaches of the Internet in search of new facts to weave into my narrative. In a sense, I start each morning by wondering what I am going to say on my screen today.

What Is Most Frustrating About Being a Medical Writer?

Probably each medical writer would answer this question a little differently. For me it is that other people—non-writers, that is—don't take the work of writing seriously. When you are hard at work composing the next paradigm-shifting medical paper, your colleagues think nothing of barging in to ask a question. The more sensitive ones ask "Are your interruptible?" before plunging ahead with what they have to say. Would they, in the same manner, recklessly disrupt a doctor-patient consultation, a teacher's conference with a student, or a surgical operation? No, they would not. But somehow, the writer's concentration on the work at hand seems fair game.

What About the Loneliness of Being a Writer?

"Nearly all works of creative originality are conceived in states of constructive alone-ness. In fact, only the creative person who is not afraid of this constructive loneliness will have command over the productive emanations of his creative mind," writes Frieda Fromm-Reichman [39]. I like the phrase "constructive aloneness," which combines the creativity of writing with the single-person nature of the work.

Undoubtedly writing is a solitary activity, but not necessarily a lonely one. It helps to have a writing partner. By this I am not necessarily describing a coauthor. Instead, I am referring to a writing partner who serves as the occasional researcher and source of bright ideas, the ever-ruthless critic, eagle-eyed proofreader, and sometimes the writer's creative muse.

For many writers, this writing partner has been the spouse. Here are some exam-ples. Albert Einstein worked closely with his first wife, Mileva Maric Einstein, and some have suggested that she was the source of the idea of relativity, or at least did the math; in any case, Albert refers in one of his letters to her to "our" work on rela-tive motion, and as part of the Einstein divorce agreement Mileva received the cash award from Albert's Nobel Prize [40, 41].

Some of Zelda Fitzgerald's words are found in Scott's writing, and his are found in hers. Patricia-Alma Hitchcock played a substantial role in production of her husband, Alfred's, films. Irving Stone's wife, Jean, researched his work and "shortened and cleaned up the manuscripts she sometimes described as verbose" [42]. James Michener's wife, Mari, was his "working partner" for decades [43].

And my wife, Anita D. Taylor, author of *How to Choose a Medical Specialty* [44], was able to dig into her remarkably diverse files and promptly provide me with the documents to support the previous two paragraphs. In addition, she is the source of my knowledge of the MBTI and my inclusion above of personality factors in writing. In the end, she will proofread every word of this book. That's what I mean by a "writing partner."

What About Other Things in Life That Compete with Writing?

One of my favorite quotes about leadership comes from a little book titled *The Leadership Secrets of Attila, the Hun:* "If you want to be a leader, you need to want it badly, because leading takes a lot of effort" [45]. It is the same with writing, at least being a serious writer. You need to commit mental energy and, as odd as this may seem, the physical effort to sit and interact with a computer for hours on end.

I sometimes wonder how many serious medical writers, or writers of any kind, are skilled golfers, dedicated gardeners, or gourmet cooks. I suspect not many. The high-wire artist Karl Wallenda once said, "Being on the wire is living; everything else is waiting." This is how many writers feel about writing.

How Is Being a Medical Writer Like Being a Surgeon?

Surgeons are born to cut and sew. From an early age, they somehow sense their destiny, even though as children they may not understand implications of the life they will later seek. Then, when finally trained and turned loose on the public, a surgeon would rather operate than do anything else. A medical school dean once told me, "I would not really need to pay the surgeons. They would operate for nothing, just for the exhilaration of being in the operating room." Well, I think writers are much the same. From an early age, they are likely to read and write eagerly. They love what they do, and couldn't see themselves in any other occupation. If they didn't need income to pay for food, clothing, and shelter, most would write even if not paid.

But it is really heartwarming to be paid for what we do.

References

1. DeAngelis C. Quoted in: AMA manual of style: a guide for authors and editors. 10th ed. New York: Oxford University Press; 2007.
2. Jenner E. An inquiry into the causes and effects of the variolae vaccinae. London: Sampson Low; 1798.
3. Edward Jenner book. http://commons.wikimedia.org/wiki/File:Edward_Jenner_book.jpg.
4. Semmelweis I. The etiology, the concept, and the prophylaxis of childbed fever. Madison, WI: Univ Wisconsin Press; 1983.
5. Garrison F. An introduction to the history of medicine. Philadelphia: Saunders; 1913.
6. Johnson WM. The true physician: the modern "doctor of the old school". New York: Macmillan; 1936.
7. Marshall B. The pathogenesis of non-ulcer dyspepsia. Med J Aust. 1985;143:319.
8. Smith R. The trouble with medical journals. Med Leg J. 2008;76:79.
9. Hoven AD. New models of health-care delivery. Wall St J. 2014;30. http://online.wsj.com/news/articles/SB20001424052702304518704579522040414884208.
10. Kean S. The tale of the dueling neurosurgeons. Boston: Little, Brown; 2014.
11. Woodrow R. The life of a medical writer. http://www.slideshare.net/woodrowr/the-life-of-a-medical-writer-tips-for-people-considering-a-medical-writing-career.
12. Iniesta I. Hippocratic corpus. BMJ. 2011;342:688.
13. Hippocrates Rubens. This image is in the public domain. http://commons.wikimedia.org/wiki/File:Hippocrates_rubens_cropped.jpg.
14. Simmons JG. Doctors and discoveries: lives that created today's medicine. Boston: Houghton Mifflin; 2002.

15. Strathem P. A brief history of medicine: from Hippocrates to gene therapy. New York: Running Press; 2005.
16. Rosner F. The medical legacy of Moses Maimonides, a prominent medieval physician. Einstein Quart J Biol Med. 2002;19:125.
17. Thomas Sydenham engraving. This image is in the public domain. http://commons.wikimedia. org/wiki/Thomas_Sydenham#mediaviewer/File:Sydenham.jpg.
18. The works of Thomas Sydenham MD. Greenhill WA, editor. London: Sydenham Society; 1844.
19. Golden R. A history of William Osler's The principles and practice of medicine. Osler Library studies in the history of medicine No. 8. Montreal: McGill University; 2004.
20. Cuneiform writing. http://www.hu.mtu.edu/~scmarkve/2910Su11/WrSys/ evolofcuneiform3100-600BC.htm.
21. Edwin Smith papyrus. This image is in the public domain because the copyright has expired. http://commons.wikimedia.org/wiki/File:Edwin_Smith_Papyrus_v2.jpg.
22. Velshi A. The Internet is just warming up. Money. 2013;3:30.
23. What is the oldest scientific journal? http://casesblog.blogspot.com/2008/10/what-is-oldest-scientific-journal.html.
24. Philosophical Transactions of the Royal Society, Volume I, 1665 and 1666. This image is in the public domain because the copyright has expired. http://commons.wikimedia.org/wiki/ File:Philosophical_Transactions_-_Volume_001.djvu.
25. How many science journals? Sci Intell InfoPros. http://scienceintelligence.wordpress. com/2012/01/23/how-many-science-journals/.
26. Sivasubramanian H, et al. "Not always a Baker's Cyst" – an unusual presentation of a central voluminous postero-medial meniscal cyst. Open Ortho J. 2012;6:589. http://www.ncbi.nlm. nih.gov/pmc/articles/PMC3468909/.
27. Asfar P, et al. High versus low blood-pressure target in patients with septic shock. N Engl J Med. 2014;370:1581.
28. The Cochrane Collaboration. About us. http://www.cochrane.org/about-us.
29. Theodoratou E, et al. Vitamin D and multiple health outcomes. BMJ. 2014;348:2035.
30. Bazerman C. The informed writer: using sources in the disciplines. 5th ed. New York: Houghton-Mifflin; 1995. http://writing.colostate.edu/textbooks/informedwriter/.
31. Writers according to Myers-Briggs. http://youngbloodblog.wordpress.com/myersbriggs/.
32. DiTiberio JK, Hammer AL. Introduction to type in college. Mountain View, CA: CPP, Inc.; 1993.
33. Jensen GH, DiTiberio JK. The MBTI and writing blocks. Gainesville, FL: MBTI News; 1983. p. 14.
34. Stegner W. Quoted in: Asimov. How to enjoy writing. New York: Walker and Co.; 1987. p. 134.
35. O'Reilly B, et al. Killing Kennedy: the end of Camelot. New York: Macmillan; 2012.
36. Diagnostic and statistical manual of mental disorders, 5th ed. Arlington, VA: American Psychiatric Association Publishing, 2013.
37. Frances A. DSM-5 writing mistakes will cause great confusion. Huff Post Sci. 2014. http:// www.huffingtonpost.com/allen-frances/dsm5-writing-mistakes-wil_b_3419747.html.
38. Adams DH, et al. Transcatheter aortic-valve replacement with a self-expanding prosthesis. N Engl J Med. 2014;370:1790.
39. Fromm-Reichman F. Loneliness. Washington, DC: W.A. White Psychiatric Foundation; 1969.
40. Einstein's wife: the life of Mileva Maric Einstein. http://www.pbs.org/opb/einsteinswife/ science/womenscience.htm/.
41. Did Einstein's first wife secretly coauthor his 1905 relativity paper? MIT Technol Rev. http://www.technologyreview.com/view/427621/did-einsteins-first-wife-secretly-coauthor-his-1905-relativity-paper/.
42. Oliver M. Prolific biographical novelist Irving Stone dies. Oregonian. August 27, 1989.
43. Wohler M. Peripatetic Michener doesn't let age get in the way. Oregonian. July 12, 1986.
44. Taylor AD. How to choose a medical specialty. 5th ed. Minneapolis, MN: Mill City Press; 2012.
45. Roberts W. Leadership secrets of Attila the Hun. New York: Grand Central Publishing; 1989.

Chapter 2
Getting Started in Medical Writing

This chapter is about some early steps on a medical writing journey. Even if you consider yourself a somewhat experienced writer, some of the insights and tips in this chapter may prove helpful. For example, have you given much thought to the time of day you write, about your writing environment, and about your writing "toolbox?" Maybe there are writing opportunities you have not considered, such as letters to the editor, that can advance your career. Should you write for a local newspaper, or perhaps create a blog site?

As is the case with many of the stories in this book, we medical writers can learn a lot from the experiences of professional writers in all fields, including novelists, poets, and playwrights, as well as backstories such as the identity of the physician who was the inspiration for Sir Arthur Conan Doyle's character Sherlock Holmes and where J.K. Rowling penned the first of the Harry Potter novels.

Why Should I Write?

An article by Daguara reports what 100 authors had to say about why they write. Here are the top categories of responses [1]:

- Of these respondents, 15 % reported writing as a way to express themselves. One author reported, "It's a great outlet for expression. I often wake up in wee hours of the morning with story ideas that it would impossible for me not to write. The ideas will keep nagging me until I get them written down."
- Thirteen percent state that they write because they have to. "It's who I am. It's what I love. I even write for fun on top of writing for a living. I couldn't NOT write. I need to write like I need to breathe, to eat, it's vital to me."
- Helping others is why 13 % of writers write, which Daguara describe as "the clearest reason as to why writers write."
- Eleven percent of respondents reported writing to educate. One author tells, "It's the academic in me."

© Springer International Publishing Switzerland 2015
R.B. Taylor, *What Every Medical Writer Needs to Know*,
DOI 10.1007/978-3-319-20264-8_2

The responses reported above are from writers, in general. What about medical school faculty members? The professional academician, who needs to develop a promotion-worthy curriculum vitae, knows the importance of writing, and specifically of the high value of research articles published in peer-reviewed journals. Thus if you ask an assistant professor of medicine to identify the reasons why he or she writes, career advancement would be high on the list.

How much do publications matter in academic career advancement? One informative study describes academic promotion at Johns Hopkins University School of Medicine. The authors report, "Those who were promoted had had about twice as many articles published in peer-reviewed journals as those who were not promoted" [2].

Another study by Beasley et al. compares clinician-educators (CEs), who typically focus on teaching rather than writing, and clinician-investigators (CIs), whose job description emphasizes research and publication. Here is what they found regarding promotion of 604 internal medicine junior faculty: "The unadjusted sixth-year promotion rate for CEs was 16 %, while for CIs it was 26 % ($P=0.002$)" [3]. Simply stated, at the same length of time on faculty, the clinician-educator was much less likely to be promoted compared with the clinician-investigator.

What about the medical communicator, the person who writes for a living in science or industry, producing monographs, proposals, white papers, brochures, reports, patient education materials, and more? These people may be the luckiest of all. They get to do what they love—write—and get paid for it. Most of us write as an avocation; we write, but clinical practice, teaching, research, or administration is our day job. The medical communicator is the true professional medical writer.

How Do I Get Started If I Have Never Had Anything Published?

Seeking a guide who has walked the trail is a good way to begin. The neophyte, but aspiring, medical writer should seek an experienced mentor, someone who has a number of publications in the area in which he or she would like to write: research report, review article, book chapter, or even, eventually, an authored book. Look for someone who is willing to give you some pointers and to look over your work as things progress. An experienced mentor can be very helpful in navigating the submission process. Sometimes an experienced writer will invite a promising young, would-be author to collaborate on a project. Even if this means that you will do most of the work, the experience will be invaluable, and you will notch a publication on your curriculum vitae, although you may not be the first author.

There are specific opportunities and model the tenderfoot medical writer should consider. Several of these are described below; but first here are some examples from history.

How Did Some Famous Writers, Including Medical Writers, Get Started?

Every medical writer has a first published work. It may be an article, a book chapter, or a memoir. With that accomplishment came the "writer's itch," the urge to put more words on blank pages, that can only be relived by the "scratch of the pen" or, today, by the tap of computer keys. Here are some anecdotes about how a selection of notable (more or less, in some cases) medical writers got started.

In 1872, general practitioner George Huntington penned the first comprehensive description of a hereditary disorder with choreiform movements, psychiatric manifestations, and progressive cognitive impairment. It described the observations of Huntington and his physician father and grandfather of several generations of a family living in East Hampton on Long Island, New York. Published in the *Medical and Surgical Reporter of Philadelphia*, the report was Huntington's first paper [4] (see Fig. 2.1). He was just 22 years old, and had received his MD degree only the year before. Today we call the disorder Huntington disease. During his long career as a physician, Huntington published just one subsequent scientific paper.

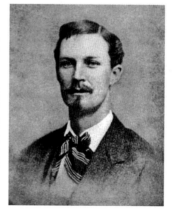

Fig. 2.1 George Huntington and his article "On Chorea," 1872 [43]

Fig. 2.2 Abraham
Verghese, author of *My
Own Country: A Doctor's
Story* [44]

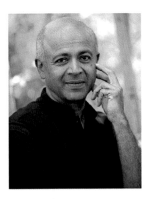

When Sir Arthur Conan Doyle attended the University of Edinburgh, he was a classmate of Robert Louis Stevenson and James Barrie, all of whom would go on to be famous authors. Doyle's writing career began while he was in medical school, with a short story set in South Africa, *The Mystery of Sasassa Valley* [5]. He went on to author the immensely popular Sherlock Holmes series, with his intrepid detective hero based on one of his professors at the University of Edinburgh Medical School, Doctor Joseph Bell.

Out of necessity to pay for his tuition, Anton Chekhov also began writing while in medical school. His first works were tales of everyday life in Russia, authored under various pseudonyms. One of Chekhov's pen names was "Man Without a Spleen."

W. Somerset Maugham's first book was a biography of opera composer Giacomo Meyerbeer, but it was his second book *Liza of Lambeth*, based on his experiences as a physician, that became highly lucrative and prompted Maugham to change careers from medicine to writing [6].

We remember Elisabeth Kübler-Ross for her 1969 book *On Death and Dying,* which elucidates the five stages of grief: denial, anger, bargaining, depression, and acceptance [7]. This book evolved from a series of seminars about terminal patients presented at the University of Chicago Pritzker School of Medicine. Following the success of her groundbreaking book, Kübler-Ross went on to write other works on the general topic of dying and death.

Abraham Verghese's first book, *My Own Country: A Doctor's Story*, tells of a young doctor beginning practice in Johnson City, Tennessee, in the mid-1980s who noted a number of patients with similar, progressive disease manifestations unresponsive to his best therapeutic efforts [8]. This was the time medicine was beginning to recognize a new disease: acquired immunodeficiency syndrome (AIDS). Initially the disease seemed to be most prevalent in homosexual men, drug users, or Haitian immigrants, certainly not the typical residents of rural Tennessee. Verghese, inspired by the courage of his patients and the prejudice, sometimes abandonment, they faced, penned a book that launched his successful writing career (see Fig. 2.2).

Indian-America Surgeon Atul Gawande, author of *Complications: A Surgeon's Notes On An Imperfect Science* [9], began writing during his surgery residency, when a friend who was editor of an online magazine *Slate*, asked him to submit an article telling about the world of the surgical resident.

As for me, my medical writing career began when, a few years after I entered private practice in a small town in upstate New York, I wrote an article about my office practice, never indexed and now long-lost, published in *Medical Economics* magazine. Nine years and three books later, I was invited to edit one of the two major reference books in my specialty of family medicine [10].

What Models Offer Early Writing Opportunities for Aspiring Medical Writers?

Many medical students and residents, by serving as part-time laboratory assistants, manage to get their names listed a coauthors on reports of basic science research. These publications may flesh out their curriculum vita and residency or fellowship applications, even though a report on amino acids in rat livers rarely has much relevance to the young physicians' future specialty choices. Although the papers are almost never composed by the medical student or resident assistants, the experiences offer an early glimpse into the process of medical writing.

Then the young professional, having finished medical school and residency, or perhaps a doctor of philosophy program, embarks on a medical writing path. The following are some ways to gain valuable experience and to feel the joy of seeing your name in print.

Letter to the Editor

Many current writers' publication lists begin with a letter to the editor. For me, during my novice years in academics, it was a letter to the *Journal of the American Medical Association* (JAMA), commenting on an article about hypertension detection and management [11]. I think that this early success gave me courage to try more demanding models of medical writing.

Today, however, most items in the "Letters" section of the major medical journals are submitted by well-funded research teams commenting on the published works of other well-funded research teams, generally from internationally known institutions. In response to an article about stenting for renal-artery stenosis [12], the *New England Journal of Medicine* (NEJM) published responses from a number of prestigious institutions including Aristotle University in Greece, George Washington University in Washington, DC, Tokyo Heart Institute, Ochsner Medical Center in New Orleans, Cardiovascular Center Aalst in Belgium, the University of Catania in Italy, and others.

According to the International Association of Scientific, Technical, and Medical Publishers (STM), there are some 28,000 active scholarly peer-reviewed journals published [13]. Most of us subscribe to several of these publications, or receive them gratis, thanks to the advertiser support or as a benefit of our dues to a professional organization. Almost all encourage readers to submit letters commenting on articles published, and hence the opportunities to publish a letter are enormous.

An example of one special way to get your comments read by others is the *British Medical Journal* (BMJ) *Rapid Response* electronic letters to the editor. Yes, you will need to actually read the BMJ to comment on an article, but this journal has been one of the most egalitarian, yet scholarly, of all medical publications. Letters to be published in the main weekly journal are selected from the Rapid Responses, and the individual reader has a fair chance of having comments considered. To submit a comment to BMJ Rapid Response, find the article on bmj.com. Then click on "Send a Response," and paste your comment into the box titled "Compose your Response." Full instructions are found at the bmj.com website [14].

Just because your "target" journal rejects your letter doesn't mean that it can't be submitted elsewhere. A few years ago, I wrote a report documenting how the manufacturer of a certain pain medication was making claims in an advertisement in JAMA that were supported only by a single, slightly suspicious, unpublished poster. After its rejection by JAMA, my report was published as a Letter in *Family Medicine* [15]. The published letter was longer than the original submission to JAMA, and told the rejection story plus some musings about the influence of the pharmaceutical industry on what is and is not published in our respected journals.

Newsletter

Not all articles on medical topics are published by journals and magazines. There are many online newsletters that welcome well-written practice insights. One of these is *Kaiser Health News*. A recent post by Roni Caryn Rabin was titled "15-Minute Visits Take a Toll on Doctor-Patient Relationship." In this piece Rabin quotes one source as saying, "Doctors have one eye on the patient and one eye on the clock." She holds that rushed doctors listen less, even though "making the patient feel they have been heard may be one of the most important elements of doctoring" [16].

While on the topic of newsletters, if you are in a private practice and still send out paper bills to patients, consider enclosing a newsletter with your monthly statement. You might write about the importance of childhood immunizations, first-aid tips, flu shots, when to call the doctor, or diseases you are seeing in the office that season.

Research Letter

JAMA publishes what it calls Research Letters, which Zylke calls, "smaller but fully functional cousins of the larger and flashier model" [17]. These submissions should follow the IMRaD model of Introduction, Methods, Results, and Discussion, but must do so in 600 words or less, and contain no more than six reference citations. JAMA Research Letters are cited in PubMed and may receive citations in other articles. If you and your colleagues have performed a well-designed study, but not a million-dollar blockbuster multicenter research epic with a catchy acronym, then the Research Letter may be your ideal venue for publication.

I use JAMA as an example because of its clear pathway to submission. Other journals also publish many research reports and other types of investigation as "letters." Increasingly, authors submitting papers for publication are receiving responses stating that the submitted articles are too long to be published as submitted, but will be considered if shortened to 500 words and re-submitted as letters.

Case Report

Even the physician who has not penned an essay since college sometimes recognizes a unique case that has significance for other clinicians. Writing up this observation, perhaps documenting findings with photographs, and submitting it to the right journal can yield a satisfying publication. As an example of a case report that told of a previously unrecognized disease, adiposis dolorosa was first described by Dercum in a report of three cases published in 1899; today the disease bears his name—Dercum disease [18].

Over the years, the case report, sometimes called a "brief report," has been an important part of the medical literature, sometimes serving as the sentinel alert to the presence of a new disease. The emergence of Middle East respiratory syndrome (MERS) was described in an NEJM "brief report" by an Egyptian virologist in 2012 [19]. The worldwide risks of this newly described illness are currently being debated.

The "big four" medical journals—NEJM, JAMA, BMJ, and *The Lancet*—all publish case reports from time to time. So do many subspecialty journals. If you have observed a fascinating case, or perhaps a curious cluster of cases, consider writing a case report. Consulting the Instructions for Authors of your favorite journal will tell if they publish case reports.

Personal Observations and Meaningful Anecdotes

JAMA publishes a regular feature titled "A Piece of My Mind." Recently Michael B. Rothberg contributed an essay titled "The $50,000 Physical," telling how some incidental findings on his father's routine physical examination led to a train wreck of further testing, interventions, and complications culminating in a huge medical bill and, paradoxically, the reassurance that there had been nothing seriously wrong in the first place [20].

The journal *Family Medicine* printed an essay by David Evans telling of his feelings when a former patient called to report having her fourth child. In "What Patients Give Us: One Story of the Doctor-Patient Relationship," he describes how he had delivered this patient's first three babies. Then he left his private practice and entered academic medicine. Now Evans is happy for the birth of a healthy baby, but is sad because he was not present for the event. In reflecting on his transition from practitioner to educator, he writes, "What I wasn't ready for was the challenge of leaving the deep, time-tested relationships I had developed with my patients" [21].

If you have an insight like those I just described, consider writing it up for publication. This is one arena in which being a faculty member at a medical school or having National Institutes of Health (NIH) grant funding offers no advantage in seeking publication.

Writing for a Newspaper

Just in passing, I will suggest that your local newspaper might welcome a pertinent letter from you. The word of the health professional carries weight, and will get extra attention when the editorial staff is considering which letters to publish. You may choose to comment on a public health issue in the community or the need for increased health services in some area. Especially important may be your comments regarding the issues linking medicine and politics. The next time you disagree with an article, editorial, or letter about the Affordable Care Act, Medicaid expansion, health care costs, or some other facet of how health care is delivered, consider penning a response. If we health professionals remain silent about what is happening in health economics and political decisions, we have only ourselves to blame if we don't like the outcomes. Local newspaper Letters to the Editor columns are a great way to make your views known.

Blog Site

One way to get some practice writing about medicine is to start your own blog. Other than the reasons stated above for writing in the first place, why might you "blog?"

One reason is to become known, that is, to attract patients or referrals. Or perhaps you have written a book you want to publicize. Whatever your reason, creating and maintaining a blog site can be fun.

There are a number of blog sites you could visit to see models of success. One is Kevinmd, the blog of Kevin Pho, MD, who describes his site as "social media's leading physician voice" [22]. Recent posts included thoughts titled "Have ADHD diagnoses reached a tipping point?" and "How Bingo kept a patient going."

A more humorous blog site is drgrumpy, more specifically Doctor Grumpy in the House [23]. In a post, Doctor Grumpy takes on wordy nonsense such as this statement: "A database, in this case big data, provided the foundation for the potential to use-state-of-art analytics to generate truly actionable insights." Doctor G. asks: "WTF does that mean?" And there is also a record of fanciful dialogue titled "Medicine by Committee."

According to *Forbes* magazine, the best doctor blog on the Internet is written by a South African surgeon under the name Bongi [24]. The website is titled *Other Things Amanzi*, with the heading, "The thoughts of a surgeon in the notorious province of Mpumalanga, South Africa comments on the private and state sector, but mostly my personal journey through surgery" [25]. Here I read of a heavy-drinking, heavy-smoking female patient with an active bleeding ulcer who seems to find her physician attractive and is disappointed to find that he is married. One reader of the blog responded to Dr. Bongi, "You had an opportunity to improve the gene pool, and you didn't take it! Very funny story …."

Among the many other medical blogs are DB's Medical Rants (medrants.com), The Derm Blog (thedermblog.com), and Blog, MD: Musings of a Pediatric Hematologist-Oncologist (http://blogmd.samblackman.org/). The good news about blogs (or maybe it is the bad news) is that no editor will tinker with your cunningly crafted phrases or witty narrative. What you write goes out for all to see.

Medical blogging has become so popular that the realm has a name: the Medblogosphere. There are awards for the *Best Medical/Health Issues* blog. One is by *Best Health* magazine [26]. For those who want to begin a medical blog, a useful place to start is the website "How to Start Your Medical Blog: An Introduction to the Medblogosphere" [27].

What Should I Write About?

Peter Lynch, the manager who propelled Fidelity's Magellan Fund to record heights (a 29 % average annual return from 1977 to 1990), is famous for advising, "Invest in what you know." The concept was called *local knowledge*. Using this philosophy, if you know about fashion, consider buying stock in clothing and shoe companies; if you know about cars, investigate car manufacturers; if your expertise is travel, study the balance sheets of hotels and restaurants.

The same philosophy holds for medical writing. Write about what you know. Just having a health professional degree doesn't make you an expert on everything, but you do have credibility when writing about what you do every day. The case reports, personal observations, and blog site writings above serve as examples.

Here is what Kurt Vonnegut, author of *Slaughterhouse-Five* and other novels, recommends: "Find a subject you care about and which you in your heart feel others should care about. It is this genuine caring, and not your games with language, which will be the most compelling and seductive element in your style. I am not urging you to write a novel, by the way—although I would not be sorry if you wrote one, provided you genuinely cared about something. A petition to the mayor about a pothole in front of your house or a love letter to the girl next door will do" [28].

Should I Write About My Patient Care Experiences?

Sooner or later, and especially during the early years of retirement, most doctors are tempted to write a book about the interesting cases they have encountered during a lifetime of practice. In fact, many such books are penned, and some are quite compelling reading. Here are two of them:

The Adventures of Dr. Huckleberry, by E. R. Huckleberry, MD, is the story of the author's practice in the seaside town of Tillamook, Oregon, in the early twentieth century [29]. A local physician gave me a copy of the book in 1984, shortly after I agreed to take a medical school faculty position in Oregon, moving there from the East Coast; I think he wanted me to know what medical practice in Oregon was really about. In the book there are stories of logging camps and the lumber mill, and all the attendant injuries. But this is the tale of a generalist physician and life in his community, including home visits, "fishermen's boils," and dealing with elk in the strawberry patch. The book's copyright is held by the Oregon Historical Society, which I believe underwrote its publication.

Another example is *A Country Doctor's Casebook: Tales from the North Woods*, by Roger A. MacDonald, MD [30]. In this book, we read of the medical adventures of Miss Cora Benson, who "stood straight as a tall pine"; Pudge Dalafus in the emergency room with a face full of windshield glass fragments from an auto accident; and Roxie Bascolm, who reported, "I got pains down there and my monthlies won't quit." The book's publication was supported in part by the George W. Nielson Fund, and published by Borealis Books, an imprint of the Minnesota Historical Society Press.

The books by Doctors Huckleberry and MacDonald, intriguing as they are, highlight the two problems with this type of book; the first is patient confidentiality. No matter how many years have passed, patients and their families recall memorable medical events. As the author of a practice retrospective, just imagine getting a phone call from a patient who, long ago, you treated for a communicable disease acquired during a weekend in Las Vegas, or a single mother whose neglect of her child prompted a call to Child Protective Services, all detailed in your book. Changing names of those involved cannot erase patient and family recollections of what happened. The sort of events I just described is typical of the scenarios likely to be described in books about "interesting cases from my career as a physician." As part of the huge confidentiality problem presented, I think there is a significant litigation risk.

The second issue with such books is one of readership. There is not a ready audience of readers waiting to peruse the pages of your case narratives. Note that both books described above relied on outside funding—historical societies—to achieve publication. This means that, if you do write the story of your years in practice, you will embark upon a probably fruitless search for a commercial publisher. Or you will decide to self-publish the book, as described in Chap. 5.

What Tools Does a Writer Need?

If answering this question a decade ago, I would have described the need for a computer with Internet access, a sheath of pencils, and a good medical dictionary. Today, everyone has a computer, and probably also a tablet and smartphone; we live our lives electronically "connected." Now if I want to know the meaning of a word such as "kakidrosis" or "horripilation," I don't reach for a six-pound dictionary. Instead I type the word in the Google search box, and up comes a site with the definition, and even the etymology of the word. And on today's desktop (the horizontal one, not the computer screen), pencils and erasers are often just anachronistic dust catchers.

What the medical writer really needs, then and now, is a clear idea of what needs to be said and how it will be organized. I will tell more about this as we go along.

Is There a Best Time of Day to Write?

Some writers are larks; others are owls. For example, Charles Dickens was an early-bird writer. He sat at his desk, writing assiduously, from 9 a.m. until early afternoon. From then on he walked, quietly pondering what he had put on paper in the morning hours [31]. Maya Angelou and Ernest Hemingway also wrote in the morning. In contrast, Robert Frost, was a late-in-the day writer, who usually arose about noon, started work later in the afternoon, and then often wrote into the wee hours of the morning [32].

Of course, for Dickens and Frost, writing was their day job. Today's medical writer, unless employed professionally by industry, often writes when the opportunity presents itself—before the family awakes in the morning, between meetings, after the last patient is seen, or while the family watches television in the evening.

Based on a poll of writers, Wightman offers an interesting theory about what times of day are best to undertake various aspects of writing: Mornings are best for problem solving; create your outline during the "lark" hours. Afternoons, especially "between noon and 2 p.m. … when your blood circulation increases, verbal reasoning is increased, and mental alertness is sustained," are the best time to be productive, to get a lot of words on the screen. Evening is for creativity; being at your least alert state of mind ("groggy") allows your brain to engage in creative insight [33].

Perhaps "evening creativity" fits the biorhythms of many of the writers surveyed, but after lunch my mental alertness tends to ebb—until I have had a power nap. In the end, my best advice is to write at the best time for you according to your competing demands and personal biorhythms.

I found one interesting study of various writers and the times they arose to begin work in the morning. For example, James Joyce and F. Scott Fitzgerald were mid-morning risers while Sylvia Plath and Oliver Sacks were up before sunrise. The author of the study, Maria Popova, found that authors who arose early in the morning were more likely to win awards, and those who began their day later in the morning tended to be more prolific [34].

What About Where I Write?

Famous authors have written in some interesting places. Robert Frost wrote in his rustic cabin in Vermont. Marcel Proust's writing space was a cork-lined room [33]. Agatha Christie often wrote while sitting in a huge bathtub, while Gertrude Stein did some of her best writing in the seat of her Model T automobile. Maya Angelou often wrote in a hotel room, but insisted upon removal of all art from the walls: she wanted nothing to divert attention from the work at hand [35]. J.K. Rowling wrote *Harry Potter and the Philosopher's Stone*—in pencil—sitting at a table in Nicolson's cafe in Edinburgh [36].

Medical writers are generally more pragmatic about where they write. Few of us have the luxury of a soundproof room, a huge tub, or a cozy cafe. For us, the workspace is likely to be the work or home office, often both at different times. What most of us really need is reasonable lighting, an up-to-date computer with lightning-quick Internet access, and relative freedom from distractions.

Can I Make a Living as a Freelance Medical Writer?

A professional medical writer can earn a good salary. One site reports that the median medical writer salary in the USA is $70,951 [37]. Freelance medical writing is another story.

Being a freelance medical writer sounds liberating and exciting. Imagine being in control of your hours, your income, and your professional destiny. But being a freelance medical writer seems a tough way to make a living.

I visited a website titled *Freelancer: Medical Writing Jobs* [38]. On the date of my search (Summer of 2014) the website described "6314 Medical Writing Jobs to Date"; presumably that many jobs had been brokered through "Our Medical Writing Community." Here I found several writing projects posted; freelance writers are invited to bid.

One of the posted projects was headed, "Medical Writer Needed." The job described required the following skills: "Articles, medical writing, article rewriting." The text went on to state, "I am looking for an experienced medical writer who can write articles and descriptions within given timeframe." The "price" offered: $2 per hour. One freelancer had actually bid on this job, but was asking for "$3 per hour."

Perhaps I had looked at the wrong website. I tried another titled "oDesk Corporation" [39]. Here I found a post: "Medical Article Writers Required on Urgent Basis." The specifics of the offer are as follows: "We require high quality medical writer for writing the high quality articles. Newbies will be preferred. We pay 4 dollars per article of 1000 words." This is a "fixed-price" offer with a budget of $80. To put the payment in perspective, this chapter (Chap. 2 of the book) has about 6000 words. This means that if I wrote an article with the same word count as this chapter, I would receive the grand sum of $24 (6000 words at a rate of $4 per 1000 words). And this is before taxes.

Did I pick only the most parsimonious postings from the websites? I went back to the oDesk Corporation site and found:

- An offer of $5 to proofread a 755-word article "Amigdalite."
- A writer needed urgently for a project paying $1 per 100 words.
- A need for four short articles for a foot care newsletter: estimated budget $18.
- A high-quality writer needed for "3×500 words on dental topics." Estimated budget of $6.

- And here is a really generous job offer: "We need a high quality medical article writer on urgent basis. The articles will be from 1000 to 1500 words. We will pay 3–5 dollars per article."

I don't know a teenage baby sitter who would work for these wages.

Considering that it takes both a solid education and considerable ability to be a medical writer, these offered payments strike me as ridiculously low. From what I have learned, if you like a decent lifestyle and enjoy eating regularly, I would not advise a career as a freelance medical writer. If you, however, decide to follow this path, be sure to keep your day job, at least for a while.

Are There Associations of Medical Writers That Could Help My Career?

Joining an association is something to consider. The chief organization in the USA is the American Medical Writers Association (AMWA), with more than 5000 members in the USA, Canada, and 30 other countries, according to their website [40]. Membership includes a wide variety of writers, editors, and other medical communicators working in medical schools, pharmaceutical companies, hospitals, and government and nonprofit agencies. AMWA offers its members an annual conference, networking opportunities, and a continuing education program that includes distance learning. Members seeking freelance work can create a listing in the *AMWA Freelance Directory* for $75 yearly.

AMWA has 20 regional chapters across the USA and Canada. Some host area conferences, and all offer the opportunity to make contact with other medical communicators.

Should you join AMWA? The yearly professional membership cost is $170. If you live close enough to attend meetings and workshops, this may be a good investment, especially if you plan to use the Job Search site. If you are not planning to attend conferences, participate in continuing education programs, or seek work through the Job Search site, the cost of membership may not be justified.

AMWA is not the only association of medical writers. Here are some others you may consider, depending on your specialty and where you live:

European Medical Writers Association

Founded in 1989, the European Medical Writers Association (EMWA) has a thousand members in 39 countries. (A quick math calculation will bring you to the conclusion that some of these countries are not located in continental Europe.) The EMWA head office is located at Macclesfield, Cheshire, UK. The Association's journal, published by Maney Publishing, is titled *Medical Writing* [41].

Australasian Medical Writers Association

Sharing an acronym (AMWA) with the American Medical Writers Association, the Australasian Medical Writers Association has several hundred members from Australia, New Zealand, and nearby countries. The Association has an annual conference and offers a Professional Development Program [42].

Other Associations for Medical Writers

In addition to the writers' association mentioned above there are also:

- All India Medical Writers Association, founded in 2007.
- American Podiatric Medical Writers Association, part of the American Podiatric Medical Association.
- Canadian Science Writers Association, established in 1971, with 450 members, chiefly scholars, teachers, and journalists.
- The Society of Medical Writers, based in England, and publishing a twice-yearly journal, *The Writer*.
- World Association of Medical Editors, promoting cooperation among editors of peer-reviewed medical publications.

I Am an Aspiring Medical Writer But Editors Don't Seem to Like What I Submit: Should I Give Up or Keep Trying?

Few start their medical writing careers with stunning successes. When I was an aspiring young writer, trying to find a publisher for my early books, I collected a thick file of rejection letters, threatening my family that I would paper a room with them. Instead, I persevered, and today the rejection letters are aging souvenirs residing in my storage locker, and my walls are covered with framed book covers.

References

1. Daguara CJ. Why do writers write? 30 % of writers write to educate, influence, and help others. http://authorspromoter.com/why-writers-write/.
2. Batshaw ML, et al. Academic promotion at a medical school: experience at Johns Hopkins University School of Medicine. N Engl J Med. 1988;318:74.
3. Beasley BW. A time to be promoted: the prospective study of promotion in academia. J Gen Intern Med. 2006;21:123.
4. Huntington G. On chorea. Med Surg Repr Phila. 1872;26:317.
5. Doyle AC. The mystery of Sasassa Valley. Chambers' Edinburgh J. Sept 6, 1879.

6. Maugham WS. Lisa of Lambeth. London: T. Fisher Unwin; 1897.

7. Kübler-Ross E. On death and dying. New York: Macmillan; 1969.

8. Verghese A. My own country: a doctor's story. New York: Vintage; 1995.

9. Gawande A. Complications: a surgeon's notes on an imperfect science. New York: Holt; 2002.

10. Taylor RB, editor. Family medicine: principles and practice. 1st ed. New York: Springer; 1976.

11. Taylor RB. Hypertension detection and follow-up (letter). JAMA. 1980;244:1317.

12. Cooper CJ, et al. Stenting and medical therapy for atherosclerotic renal-artery stenosis. N Engl J Med. 2014;370:13.

13. Ware M, et al. The STM report: an overview of scientific and scholarly journal publishing. http://www.stm-assoc.org/2012_12_11_STM_Report_2012.pdf/.

14. Responding to articles. http://www.bmj.com/about-bmj/resources-readers/responding-articles/.

15. Taylor RB. Pharmaceutical advertisements, citations, and trust. Fam Med. 2010;42:744.

16. 15-Minute visits take a toll on doctor-patient relationship. Kaiser Health News. http://www.kaiserhealthnews.org/stories/2014/april/21/15-minute-doctor-visits.aspx?

17. Zylke JW. Research letters in JAMA: small but mighty. JAMA. 2013;310:589.

18. Dercum FX. Three cases of a hitherto unclassified affection resembling in its grosser aspects obesity, but associated with special nervous symptoms-adiposis dolorosa. Am J Med Sci. 1892;104:521.

19. Zaki AM, et al. Isolation of a novel coronavirus from a man with pneumonia in Saudi Arabia. N Engl J Med. 2012;367:1814.

20. Rothberg MB. The $50,000 physical. JAMA. 2014;311:2174.

21. Evans DV. What patients give us: one story of the doctor-patient relationship. Fam Med. 2014;46:387.

22. Kevinmd. http://www.kevinmd.com/blog/.

23. Doctor Grumpy in the House. http://drgrumpyinthehouse.blogspot.com/.

24. Husten L. The best doctor blog on the internet. Forbes Pharma Health Care. 2013. http://www.forbes.com/sites/larryhusten/2013/01/25/the-best-doctor-blog-on-the-internet/.

25. Other things Amanzi. http://other-things-amanzi.blogspot.com/2010/02/crushing.html?showComment=1265899587002&m=1#c6977265348242201336/.

26. Best Health Blog Awards 2013. http://www.besthealthmag.ca/special-features/bh-blog-award/.

27. How to start your medical blog: an introduction to the medblogosphere. RX Md Marketing Solutions. http://rxmdmarketingsolutions.com/how-to-start-your-medical-blog-an-introduction-to-the-medblogosphere/.

28. Vonnegut K. How to write with style. http://peterstekel.com/PDF-HTML/KurtVonnegut advice to writers.htm.

29. Huckleberry ER. The adventures of Dr. Huckleberry. Lake Oswego, OR: Spectrum; 1970.

30. MacDonald RA. A country doctor's casebook: tales from the north woods. St. Paul, MN: Boraelis Books; 2002.

31. Tomalin C. Charles Dickens: a life. New York: Viking; 2011.

32. McCrum R. The best times to write. http://www.theguardian.com/books/booksblog/2011/oct/27/best-times-to-write/.

33. Wightman KL. The best time of day to write. http://klwightman.com/2013/05/06/best-time-of-day-to-write/.

34. Vanderkam L. What sleep habits of famous writers reveal about their productivity. http://www.fastcompany.com/3026741/work-smart/what-the-sleep-habits-of-famous-writers-reveal-about-their-productivity/.

35. Johnson CB. 13 Quirky workplaces of famous authors. Writers Digest. http://www.writersdigest.com/editor-blogs/there-are-no-rules/13-quirky-workplaces-of-famous-writers/.

36. Where writers write. Pinerst. http://www.pinterest.com/sookio/where-writers-write/.

37. Medical writer salary: United States. http://www.payscale.com/research/US/Job=Medical_Writer/Salary/.

38. Freelancer: medical writing jobs and contests: https://www.freelancer.com/jobs/Medical-Writing/1/.

39. Medical writing jobs. oDesk Corporation. https://www.odesk.com/o/jobs/browse/skill/medical-writing/.

40. American Medical Writers Association. http://www.amwa.org/about_us/.

41. European Medical Writers Association. http://www.emwa.org/EMWA/About_Us/About_EMWA/EMWA/About_Us/About_EMWA.aspx?hkey=27ce6e80-c695-4062-8c9a-a37513e83c21.

42. Australasian Medical Writers Association. http://www.wfsj.org/associations/page.php?id=262.

43. On chorea with photo. This image is in the public domain. http://commons.wikimedia.org/wiki/File:On_Chorea_with_photo.jpg.

44. Abraham Verghese © BarbiReed. Photo credit: Barbi Reed his file is licensed under the Creative Commons Attribution-Share Alike 3.0 Unported license. http://commons.wikimedia.org/wiki/File:AbrahamVerghese(c)BarbiReed.jpg.

Chapter 3
The Process of Medical Writing

The process of medical writing begins with recognizing what type of writing you are doing. Are you planning a review article, a book chapter, a personal observation, letter to the editor, or a research report? The style and structure of each are quite different. For example, a personal observation should be engagingly written with vivid examples that illustrate your message; a research report is almost the opposite, and should be factual, precise, and objective.

The structure of what you are writing also varies with the article, report, or chapter.

Possible structures include linear narration of your experience with a memorable patient, a list (such as "Five New Drugs To Treat Depression"), the "news story" style giving the facts early followed by both sides of the issue, or the time-honored model of presenting the results of a research study, described below.

Whatever structure and style you use, I recommend that you employ Rudyard Kipling's *six serving men*: "I keep six honest serving men, who taught me all I knew. Their names are What and Why and When and How and Where and Who" [1].

What About the Writing Process of Some of Our Most Famous Writers?

In the last chapter I described *when* and *where* some famous authors write. Now let's see what we medical writers can learn from the *methods* of some of the great writers of all time. Some writers are prolific, with Stephen King penning ten pages a day. Others are much less productive; James Joyce agonized over every phrase and sentence. One anecdote describes when a friend asked Joyce if he had had a good, productive day. "Yes," replied Joyce, "I wrote three sentences today" [2].

Truman Capote wrote while reclining in bed or on a sofa, even when using a typewriter. Philip Roth writes standing up, pacing as he thinks, and claiming to walk a half-mile per page written [2]. Kurt Vonnegut once described doing push-ups and sit-ups during his writing sessions. Maya Angelou twisted her hair as she wrote.

© Springer International Publishing Switzerland 2015
R.B. Taylor, *What Every Medical Writer Needs to Know*,
DOI 10.1007/978-3-319-20264-8_3

To avoid distractions, Flannery O'Connor wrote while facing the unadorned surface of her wooden dresser. Jack Kerouac described writing by candlelight, and then blowing out the candle when he was done for the night [2, 3].

Vladimir Nabokov wrote on index cards, with one novel involving 2000 cards. Susan Sontag wrote with a felt-tipped pen on legal pads. William Faulkner drank heavily while writing [3].

What can medical writers learn from all this? First of all, there is no ideal writing setting. In an interview with the *Paris Review*, E. B. White, author of *Charlotte's Web* once said: "A writer who waits for ideal conditions under which to work will die without putting a word on paper" [4]. Medical writers often have other "day jobs," such as seeing patients, teaching, or doing research. Therefore, you need to write where and when you have the opportunity.

As for writing habits, I don't recommend drinking alcohol while writing, and index cards have gone out of fashion. But pacing while thinking, removing distractions, writing while standing, or taking an occasional exercise break all seem to be reasonable options.

Should I Outline My Paper Before I Begin Writing?

The world is divided into two groups of people: the outline advocates and those who consider outlining a waste of time and keystrokes. I belong to the former group. I consider my outline to be a lifeline keeping me secured to the idea I am trying to express. I try to think first about structure, then sentences, and words.

If you are writing a report of original research, your outline is prescribed. Research data is to be submitted in the IMRaD model, an acronym that stands for *Introduction, Methods, Results, and Discussion*. Any other model of presentation invites summary rejection. In addition, many journals prescribe their own version of the IMRaD model. For example, *Annals of Internal Medicine* Information for Authors calls for these sections: Background, Objective, Design, Setting, Patients, Intervention (if any), Measurements, Results, Limitations, and Conclusions [5]. So before writing your research report, be sure to check the Instructions for Authors for your target journal.

On the other hand, if you are writing a review article or book chapter, and if no other format is prescribed or seems better for the topic, consider using the traditional outline hierarchy you learned, I hope, in your high school English class (see Table 3.1) [6].

How Can I Make My Writing Easy to Read?

"Easy reading is damn hard writing," wrote nineteenth-century American author Nathaniel Hawthorne, author of *The Scarlet Letter* and *The House of Seven Gables*. It was such a pithy aphorism that Maya Angelou and others have repeated it often [7, 8].

Table 3.1 An example of a basic outline style [6]

Article title: Approach to the patient with backache
Clinical history
History of the present illness (back pain)
Other history
Past medical history
Family history
Social history
Physical examination
Testing
Imaging
Other tests
Conclusion

Here is a suggestion to help make your writing more vigorous and easier to read. Try to write as though you were speaking. To the degree that I have been successful in this effort, I would attribute it to the way I produced my first books. In the beginning, my books were dictated, often in the car as I was driving the 18 miles from the hospital to my office. Later my typist would produce a paper copy for me to edit. In this way, I heard every word—in my voice, of course—before I ever saw it on paper.

A variation of this method is useful today. Currently we write articles and books on our computers, with a handy online thesaurus tempting us to use bigger words than needed. To help guard against writing that is hard to read, do the following: When you have finished a section of your paper, read it aloud to yourself. Does it sound the way you speak? Or does it somehow seem stilted and wordy?

Writing like we speak can come especially naturally when writing an article such as Elizabeth Fortescue's *A Piece of My Mind* article titled "Keeping the Pace." The author, a marathon runner, tells the story of learning of and dealing with her own cardiac abnormality. Her story begins [9]:

> Can you feel the pulse of an excited heart, perhaps after winning a race, or falling in love? The extra thumps and tickles, the flurry of flutters that accompany such emotional highs? I use to feel them too. I remember crossing the finish line of the Boston Marathon in 1999 …

The first sentence has 18 words and only four of them have more than one syllable. She draws you in with the image of an excited heart, a race, love, and prepares you for the stories about to come describing her arrhythmia, her pregnancy, her sinus node failure, and life with a pacemaker.

Of course, writing using the phrases and cadence we use in speaking is one thing. Organization is another. What we say to one another is often disjointed. We hop from one topic to another, and we sometimes express ourselves verbally in fits and starts. In our writing we should write as we talk, but better organized. This is how thoughtful, and sometimes ruthless, editing turns an early draft into a finished writing product that you can publish with pride.

Can I Write in the First Person in Medical Articles?

Chinese writer Lin Yutang (1895–1976) wrote, "He who is afraid to use an "I" in his writing will never be a good writer" [10]. Using "I" is the best way to take ownership of your opinions. I like to use the first person in my medical books, because it lets me "have a voice" and tell stories.

Even prestigious peer-reviewed medical journals have given the okay to use the first person in reports of scientific research. Specifically, it is acceptable to use the pronoun "we" in describing what you did to your subjects, what you found, and what you conclude. For example, in a recent *New England Journal of Medicine* report titled "Risk of Pediatric Celiac Disease According to HLA Haplotype and Country," we find many instances of first-person pronouns. The Abstract states, "We studied 6403 children ...." Under Method are the phrases "...we screened 424,788 newborns" and "We used radioligand binding assays..." The Results section begins, "As of July 31, 2013, we had performed tTG antibody testing ..." [11]. The use of first person helps make an otherwise dense research report a little more readable.

I Can Never Seem to Get Punctuation Right: Where Can I Learn About This?

Read *Eats, Shoots & Leaves*, by Lynne Truss. This is a little book about punctuation. Yes, punctuation. What's more, it is written from the British perspective. Yet, against all odds, it became a best seller in England and the USA. The title is based on an old joke that begins: "A Panda goes into a bar ...." What happens next—there are three possible scenarios—depends on the punctuation. Just to pique your interest in a book that may improve your writing, here are some sample quotes [12]:

- Railing against the inappropriate use of apostrophes (such as a sign advertising *Bananas' For Sale*), Truss writes, "Evidently there used to be a shopkeeper in Bristol who deliberately stuck ungrammatical signs in his window as a ruse to draw people into the shop; they would come in to complain, and he would then talk them into buying something" (page 66).
- Truss sees the comma as a sort of grammatical sheepdog who "tears about on the hillside of language, endlessly organizing words into sensible groups and making them stay put ..." (page 79).
- She describes another punctuation mark as follows: "The semicolon has been rightly called 'a compliment from the writer to the reader'. And a mighty compliment it is, too. The sub-text of a semicolon is, 'Now this is a hint. The elements of this sentence, although grammatically distinct, are actually elements of a single notion. I can make it plainer for you—but hey! You're a reader. I don't need to draw you a map!'" (page 124).

The wrong punctuation can change the entire meaning of a sentence, a clear danger when your book is being edited by someone who does not really understand the content of your work and is simply following editorial guidelines. Consider this sentence: "In our study we found that the cardiac arrhythmia occurred in 50 % of subjects who received the test drug." It reads quite differently when a comma is inserted after the word "subjects." The meaning of the sentence has been changed and we now learn that: "In our study we found that the cardiac arrhythmia occurred in 50 % of subjects, who received the test drug." In the latter version, the only subjects who received the test drug were those who had developed the dysrhythmia.

Here is a classic example of how punctuation changes the meanings of two sentences:

Let's eat, grandma.

Or

Let's eat grandma.

What Do I Do When I Seem to Struggle with a Sentence That Just Won't Work?

In their book *The Elements of Style*, now more than five decades old, William Strunk and E. B. White offer this advice: "When you become hopelessly mired in a sentence, it is best to start fresh; do not try to fight your way through against the terrible odds of syntax. Usually what is wrong is that the construction has become too involved at some point; the sentence needs to be broken apart and replaced by two or more shorter sentences" [13].

Consider this example, based upon an 1897 commencement speech at the University of Michigan by George Herbert Palmer titled "Self-cultivation in English" [14]:

Obviously, good English is exact English in which our words should fit our thoughts like a glove, and be neither too wide nor too tight, because if too wide they will include much vacuity beside the intended matter and if too tight, they will check the strong grasp.

Discounting the somewhat formal style of the late nineteenth century, this sentence has much to recommend it. The words are generally short and strong, and there is clear imagery in the metaphor of the glove. But reading the sentence leaves me short of breath. It has too many words and clauses. Here is what Palmer really said:

Obviously, good English is exact English. Our words should fit our thoughts like a glove, and be neither too wide nor too tight. If too wide they will include much vacuity beside the intended matter, but if too tight, they will check the strong grasp [14].

How Can I Make My Medical Writing More Vigorous?

Again Strunk and White have some strong advice: "Omit needless words. Vigorous writing is concise" [13]. For example, consider the word count in some of our most enduring prose:

The first words of the Bible, "In the beginning, God created the Heavens and the Earth," has all of ten words.

Hippocrate's admonition, "As to diseases, make a habit of two things—to help, or at least do no harm," has 17 words [15].

There are 27 words in Francis Weld Peabody's often-quoted observation, "One of the essential qualities of the clinician is interest in humanity, for the secret of the care of the patient is in caring for the patient" [16].

Lincoln's Gettysburg Address had 266 words.

The Ten Commandments are presented in 295 words.

Yes, vigorous and memorable writing does not need a lot of words.

Should I Work on One Writing Project at a Time or Try to Multitask?

Among writers of all stripes there is a lively debate as to whether you should stick to one project, soldiering through until it is done versus engaging in several writing projects at any time. Most of the votes, i.e., on websites and blogs, seem to favor maintaining multiple writing projects. One site advocates writing one article or book in the morning and revising another in the afternoon, avoiding confusion by taking advantage of the different phases in any writing project. Another writer tells of working on one project until running out of ideas, and then taking up another. Still another writer tells how working on several projects at once helps prevent boredom [17].

One writer observes (and I am going to paraphrase a little here): You can work on more than one project at a time, but make sure that you actually FINISH. It is easy to start multiple articles and follow the "New Shiny" each time an idea pops in your head. But that will never get you to the point of finishing an article, chapter, or book. Writing and finishing is hard. If you allow yourself the caprice to start a new project anytime you feel the urge, nothing will get finished [17].

On the other hand, there are those who advocate writing one project at a time. One novel writer observes, "What if I didn't abandon my current book, but worked on two at once? Can you do this? I tried, and found that I couldn't. Like most writers, I get absorbed in my characters, but just couldn't hold two sets of unique characters in my head, and feel like I could do them all justice. Even with totally different genres" [18].

Does this apply to medical writers? Can or should we undertake multiple projects, or simply focus and finish the one at hand? Granted, aside from individual patients, there are few "characters" in medical articles or book chapters. But, and especially when writing a book like this, I find I wonder if I have repeated an anecdote in two different chapters or, perhaps, contradicted myself in two different discussions.

What do I do and why? I focus on one main project at a time. Staying on task to completion helps me avoid duplicating words, facts, and even illustrations. However, most of my projects are books, and books have a rhythm of action and inactivity. First there is the preparation of a "proposal," the description of what is planned.

Based on the proposal, the publisher will make a go-or-no-go decision; for this reason I put a lot of effort into crafting the best proposal I can, even knowing that none of it will ever see print.

Then comes what always seems a very long time as the editors and publisher consider the proposal, make a decision, and, I hope, prepare a contract. This can take several months. Because I try very hard not to write a book before I have a contract, I need something else to do during this time. Enter multiple projects. This is when I may write a short article or do research for the book being considered and for future projects I might undertake.

Finally I have a signed book contract. Then, for the most part, I focus on writing the book at hand until I have a finished manuscript on its way to my editor, who reviews what I have written and dispatches it to the production office. I won't see the manuscript again until page proofs arrive. During editing and production, there is another period of slack time, more opportunity to plan ahead and perhaps work on the next proposal.

My point is this: Although I might say I work on one book at a time, I am actually collecting articles, stories, quotations, and insights for several future projects. I also will occasionally take time out to read proofs. For example, even though I am writing this book, I will take time out to review the proofs of my medical history book *On the Shoulders of Medicine's Giants* that is currently in production. When the "Medicine's Giants" proofs arrive, I will leave the "Medical Writer" manuscript and not open the file until I have finished proofreading. So am I working on one book at a time or more than one?

To gain some insight into why some people work on one writing project at time versus several, let's revisit the Myers-Briggs Personality Type Indicator (MBTI), described in Chap. 1. To review briefly, the MBTI employs dichotomous responses in four categories to describe how one gets one's energy (introvert, I, vs. extravert, E), sees the world (intuitive, N, vs. sensing, S), makes decisions about what is seen (thinking, T, vs. feeling, F), and lives his or her life (judging, J, or perceiving, P). If you are an "I," an introvert, you are more likely to prefer focusing on a single article or chapter. I tend to be one of those. If you are an "E," an extravert, your preference will be to juggle many tasks at once.

Most readers of this book will, by preference or by necessity, have several writing projects going at any one time. For you multitaskers, here are some suggestions:

- Think ahead, noting deadlines and the inevitability of interruptions.
- Aim for diversity in your various projects, so that you can keep track of what you are writing in which project.
- If possible, have your various projects at different stages: one in the research phase, one being written, and one in production.
- Pick a primary task, and designate all others as subordinate.
- If you really plan to jump back and forth between tasks, you especially should consider outlining, so that you don't lose track of where you are on the back-burner project.

- Schedule periods for rest and exercise.
- Take care of yourself. Some who say "yes" to too many opportunities sometimes forget to eat and sleep.

What About the Concept of Zonal Creativity?

One of the advantages of focusing all your attention on a single project is the increased chance that you may experience *zonal creativity*. I admit it: I created the term zonal creativity. By this I mean the mental images we experience in the twilight zone that is neither deep sleep nor being fully awake. Some have told me, "I get my best ideas in the middle of the night." These creative thoughts don't occur during deep sleep, but may occur during rapid eye movement (REM) sleep. REM sleep, occurring typically about 90 min after sleep onset and recurring during the night, is periods of increased brain activity and intense dreaming. Or, the creative zone may be the time between sleep and being fully awake. If zonal creativity occurs in the awakening phase, then I think that writers who nap have an added advantage. In essence, they have one extra awakening experience each day.

Here is an example of zonal creativity. Asimov describes the experience of German chemist August Kekule von Stradonitz in 1865 as he sought to discern the arrangement of the atoms in the chemical molecule he was studying. The answer seemed to elude him until one day, as he half-dozed on a horse-drawn bus, the atoms seemed to dance in his head, and then formed into a hexagonal ring, what we know today as the benzene ring [19] (see Fig. 3.1).

Does focusing on a single project really increase the chances of experiencing zonal creativity? Perhaps this is so. I know that some of my best word choices and concrete examples of general statements have been products of twilight alertness insights. It seems to me that having one project consuming much of your waking thought offers a better chance that a great and relevant idea may occur than if your thoughts were scattered by many efforts.

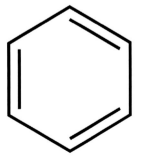

Fig. 3.1 Benzene ring, described by August Kekule von Stradonitz in 1865. Photo credit: Laurent Mazouin [20]

Do You Have Any Tips That Can Help Me Be More Efficient in My Writing?

I have three suggestions. These are methods I employ in my writing that help keep me out of trouble. They involve (1) managing references while writing my early drafts; (2) keeping track of acronyms and reference citation numbers while revising my manuscript; and (3) avoiding duplication of words, phrases, and statements in the final manuscript.

Managing References

There are reference citation management software programs. Just some of them are *EndNote*, *Bookends*, and *Biblioscape*. I don't use them, partly because they can cause problems when I submit a paper or chapter for review, and partly because of the nature of what I write.

Simply stated, if I submit a paper for editing using a reference manager software program, the editor cannot "fix" anything unless that person has (purchased) the same program. Of course, you know your target journal likes, let's say, *EndNote*. But if your paper is rejected, and you must submit it elsewhere, will the next journal use the same software program?

I first encountered this problem a few years ago when editing a large—1200+ pages—reference book. I received manuscripts from several authors who used various reference management software programs, most of which were not on my computer. It wasn't long before I added to my Instructions to Authors, "Do not prepare your manuscript using reference management software."

As to what I am writing now, most of my work involves books and book chapters. I don't write anything that has a hundred or more reference citations. Most of what I write has 20–40 references in a chapter or article, which is manageable using my favored technique. Here is what I do: When writing the first draft, I don't try to create a numbered reference list at that time. Instead I embed the reference in the draft. For example, to cite this book at this location, I would type [**Taylor RB. What every medical writer needs to know. New York: Springer; 2016**]. I type the reference in bold so that I can find it easily later. I don't add the actual reference numbers until the very end.

Then, when I am sure that the piece will have no references added to cause me to renumber all of them, I copy the citations in the text, and paste them into a nice numbered reference list.

One additional thing that I have done in recent books is to present references at the end of each section, rather than all together at the end of the chapter. I find this easier for me, with shorter lists and citations closer to the material in the text that is being referenced. I think that readers also like the reference source presented close to the fact in the text, rather than at the end of a chapter.

Keeping Track of Acronyms and Reference Citation Numbers

It is easy to duplicate acronyms and reference numbers in an article or book chapter. As I am editing my later drafts I make one "avoiding repeat acronyms/reference numbers" review of the manuscript. Here is how I do it.

As I go through the manuscript, I keep a pad of paper at hand. Each time I come to an acronym—such as AIDS or GERD—I note the use and the manuscript page number on my scratch pad. An acronym is introduced with the first use of a term; the style is acquired immunodeficiency syndrome (AIDS). After the introduction of the acronym, you can subsequently use either the full disease name or the acronym, but to use both together again would be careless.

Even worse would be to have two different items cited as, for example, reference [14] in the text. Here also I note each reference number and the page on my note pad. This is especially useful in checking when reference [14] is, by design, used several times in the text.

With this book, which has a number of figures, I will maintain a similar list of illustrations.

Avoiding Duplication of Words, Phrases, and Statements

The following may prove the most valuable of these tips. I actually create what might seem to be two drafts of the manuscript. One is the actual, true draft, created chapter by chapter. The other is a *phantom draft* of the whole manuscript, a version that will never see print, but that can help me avoid embarrassing errors.

What is in the phantom draft and why do I maintain it? In my phantom draft, I record for each chapter key words, such as *juggle* (above) and *phantom*, that I don't want to use repeatedly in the book.

Even more important is avoiding repeat reference to the same person or using the same example more than once. Thus, my phantom draft for this chapter has, in addition to "juggle" and "phantom," entries such as "Kipling six serving men," "*Eats, Shoots & Leaves*," the fact that the first sentence of the Bible has just ten words, and "zonal creativity," just to name a few.

Then as I go through later stages of editing of individual chapters, and wonder if I have used the word "phantom" too often or have told of Kipling's six serving men more than once, all I do is search my phantom draft of the entire book for the word or phrase in question. I do not need to search my true draft chapter by chapter.

How Do I Know, in the End, That My Writing Is "Working?"

One indication that your writing is "working" is, of course, that someone besides your mother and your spouse values it. Your writing is worthwhile if a journal published your article, if your employer pays you for your work, or if someone buys your book.

Your work seems to be valued if you receive a favorable letter to the editor about your article or a glowing review of your book. But what about your own assessment of your work?

I try to ask myself the following questions at the beginning of any project and also at the end:

Am I Writing Something Not Written Before?

Am I presenting some new information? The content of your writing need not be a report of a newly discovered liver enzyme or a breakthrough in the search for a cure for cancer. In many instances, the "new information" is seeing old facts in a new light. An example would be above, where I tell of Chinese writer Lin Yutang advising "He who is afraid to use an 'I' in his writing will never be a good writer." Then I relate this statement to the use of first-person pronouns in reports of scientific research.

New information can also be personal, and I try to offer this to my readers when I can. Two examples in this chapter are the *phantom draft* of a book and the concept of *zonal creativity*.

On the other hand, if I have nothing new to say, why waste my time?

Is What I Am Saying Correct?

I sometimes wish I were a novelist, rather than a medical writer. As a novelist, if my hero is in a tight spot, surrounded by hostile adversaries, I can invent a helicopter to rescue him, or she can conveniently discover a long-lost tunnel, or an earthquake can swallow the villains. I can just make stuff up. This is not the case with medical and scientific writing.

Let's say that I advised a hundred patients to eat a head of cabbage a day for a year and none of them developed cancer during that time. Have I found a way to prevent cancer? Very probably not, at least until I have secured a large grant from a neutral source (think National Institutes of Health, the NIH) and conducted a longitudinal double-blind study with a huge number of subjects and subjected my results to rigorous statistical analysis. But just such nonsense gets published every day.

No serious medical writer or academician would submit a knowingly false report. But, in an effort to build a curriculum vita and attain promotion, some medical writers seem to rush to publication with research methods that are shaky and results that are precariously supported by shaky data.

Will Anyone Care About What I Write?

For those who write for peer-reviewed journals, the review process offers one way of assessing what the scientific community—at least the reviewers who evaluate your paper—think of it. If your paper is accepted promptly with little criticism by reviewers, at least this small group of peers thinks what you have written has merit [21].

A related indication of "does anyone care?" is the *impact factor* of the journal that publishes your paper. For better or worse, journals that are most selective about what they publish tend to be those with a high impact factor. Created four decades ago by Eugene Garfield, founder of the Institute for Scientific Information, the impact factor is a calculation that is considered to indicate the relative influence of a given journal in its field. It is a numerical score, calculated annually; the higher the score, the greater the impact the journal is considered to have. If your paper is published in a high-impact journal, you might assume that it is more likely to be cited by others—an indication of its influence on the scientific community—than if it were published in a low-impact journal.

Fundamentally the score is calculated as follows: The number of times articles published in a journal during a 2-year period were cited in indexed publications during the following year (A) is divided by the total number of items published during the 2 years in question that might have been "citable" (B) [22]. Because of the method of calculation (A/B), one of the quirks of this system is that some journals circulated to a small audience can have a high impact score, even though they are not widely read.

Table 3.2 lists a sample of the widely varying impact factors for selected medical and scientific journals [23].

Yet another indication that someone values your work is whether or not what you write generates comments: letters to the editor that are published or comments offered online. Even comments that disagree with your writing should be treasured; after all, the person who commented read your article, thought about it, and cared enough to reply.

Table 3.2 Five-year impact factors for a variety of journals

Journal	Five-year impact factor
Canadian Family Physician	1.589
Cell	34.774
Clinical Science	4.181
Journal of Alzheimer Disease	4.188
Journal of the American Medical Assn.	29.684
New England Journal of Medicine	50.075
South African Journal of Surgery	0.381
World Neurosurgery	0.680

Have I Written My Article, Chapter, or Book as Well as I Can?

Even if you have conducted the study titled "Cabbage: A Factor in Cancer Prevention" (CAFCP) and demonstrated statistically that eating a head of cabbage a day keeps cancer away, if your paper is poorly written, the journal editor will send it right back to you for more work. Be kind to yourself, your reviewers, your editor, and your eventual readers. Do not submit your work until it is the best you can make it.

References

1. Kipling R. Poem following the story "Elephant's Child" in Just So Stories. CreateSpace Independent Publishing Platform; Accessed 6 Mar 2014.
2. Bargauta L. Learn from the greats: 7 writing habits of amazing writers. http://writetodone. com/learn-from-the-greats-7-writing-habits-of-amazing-writers/.
3. Massara K. Weird writing habits of famous authors. http://flavorwire.com/193101/weird-writing-habits-of-famous-authors/10.
4. White EB. The art of the essay No. 1. Paris Rev. http://www.theparisreview.org/interviews/4155/the-art-of-the-essay-no-1-e-b-white.
5. Annals of Internal Medicine Information for Authors. http://annals.org/public/authorsinfo. aspx#manuscript-preparation.
6. Taylor RB. The joys of outlining in medical writing. European Medical Writers Association. Med Writ. 2012;21:205.
7. Nathaniel Hawthorne. Brainyquote. http://www.brainyquote.com/quotes/quotes/n/nathanielh108636.html.
8. Maya Angelou interview: How I write: http://www.thedailybeast.com/articles/2013/04/10/maya-angelou-how-i-write.html.
9. Fortescue EB. Keeping the pace. JAMA. 2014;311:2383.
10. Yutang L. The importance of living. New York: Reynal & Hitchcock; 1937.
11. Liu E, et al. Risk of pediatric celiac disease according to HLA haplotype and country. N Engl J Med. 2014;371:42.
12. Truss L. Eats, shoots, & leaves. New York: Gotham; 2003.
13. Strunk Jr W, White EB. The elements of style. rev ed. New York: Macmillan; 1959.
14. Palmer GH. Self-cultivation in English, and the glory of the imperfect. New York: Crowell; 1897. p. 14–5.
15. Hippocrates. Epidemics, Book 1, Section XI.
16. Peabody FW. The care of the patient. JAMA. 1927;88:877–82.
17. Working on multiple books at the same time. http://absolutewrite.com/forums/showthread. php?t=211994.
18. Ing G. Can you write two books at once? http://www.graemeing.com/2012/10/06/can-you-write-two-books-at-once/.
19. Asimov I. Isaac Asimov's book of facts. New York: Bell; 1979. p. 99.
20. Benzene-Kekule-2D-skeletal.png. Public domain. http://commons.wikimedia.org/wiki/File:Benzene-Kekule-2D-skeletal.png.
21. Bohannon J. Who's afraid of peer review? Science. 2013;342:60. http://www.sciencemag.org/content/342/6154/60.full/.
22. The Thompson Reuters impact factor. Web Sci. http://wokinfo.com/essays/impact-factor/.
23. Impact factor list 2012. CiteFactor. http://www.citefactor.org/journal-impact-factor-list-2012. html/.

Chapter 4
Medical Writing Pointers and Pitfalls

In 40 years of medical writing, involving 34 books and several hundred papers, I have learned a few things. I have learned that having coauthors can be a mixed blessing. I have learned not to get too involved in a book project without a contract from the publisher. I have learned that a book review without a single negative comment lacks credibility. I have learned that if a paper is good and if I am persistent, it will find its way into print. I have learned that in seeking publication, the author's name, title, and institution matter, in spite of what you may be told. And that's not all.

I have also experienced a lot of misadventures. I have written articles that were too long for my target journal. I have submitted articles to inappropriate journals. I have, at times, not paid proper attention to the Instructions to Authors. And once, decades ago, in an article about innovation in medicine, I used as an example the instance in which Alexander Graham Bell, in the first telephone message in 1876, said to his assistant, "What hath god wrought!" Whoops. Those words are what Samuel F. B. Morse telegraphed in the initial demonstration of his invention in 1844 over a line from Washington DC to Baltimore, Maryland. What Graham really said was, "Mr. Watson. Come here. I want to see you." Curiously, my error survived editorial review, was printed, and prompted not a single letter of correction, testimony to either my physician readers' dearth of historical knowledge or to a lack of readers in the first place.

Thus this chapter is intended to share some pointers that may make you a better medical writer, and alert you to some pitfalls that await the unwary scribe.

© Springer International Publishing Switzerland 2015
R.B. Taylor, *What Every Medical Writer Needs to Know*,
DOI 10.1007/978-3-319-20264-8_4

What Are Some Productive Habits of Experienced, Successful Writers, Both Medical and Nonmedical?

The best writers have some things in common. Of course, not all writers we know will endorse what I say next, but many of the really successful ones will. Those that endure and prevail as medical writers (1) tend to follow instructions; (2) revise more than novice writers; (3) share drafts with colleagues, seeking comments; (4) are sometimes able to see what others do not see; and (5) write often, although not necessarily for long periods of time.

Following Instructions

Every medical and scientific journal has Instructions for Authors that are readily accessible online. Here you will find requirements and suggestions such as how to construct a title, any required components of the abstract, the technical specifications for illustrations, and any requirements peculiar to the journal. For example, the Author Instructions for the *American Journal of Cardiology* state: "Research highlights are required for this journal. Provide 3–5 bullet points that convey the core findings of the article, submitted in a separate file in the online submission system. Please use 'Highlights' in the file name. The 3–5 bullet points should each be a maximum 85 characters, including spaces" [1].

Virtually every medical journal publishes its Instructions for Authors on its website. Or, for those who like things all in one place, the Raymon H. Mulford Health Science Library in Toledo, Ohio, offers a free website with links to the Instructions for Authors of more than 6000 medical and scientific journals: http://mulford.meduohio.edu/instr.

Adherence to Author Instructions is also important in writing book chapters and books. The length of contributions is a frequent issue. Before embarking on a chapter or book project, be sure to determine the length permitted, and how many figures and tables there should be. Here is a tip. Not too long ago, "manuscript pages" meant double-spaced pages. This allowed for penciled editorial comments between the lines. Computer-generated manuscripts have changed all this, and manuscripts are now generally submitted single spaced. This change allows the opportunity for misunderstandings regarding length of submissions. Does 20 manuscript pages mean single or double spaced?

Some authors just don't read instructions, especially regarding contribution length. As a reference book editor I have had some authors send me manuscripts three or four times the contracted length. In order to avoid a book that is much too big, these manuscripts needed to be painfully pared down. In one instance an author, a giant in his field, contracted for a manuscript of 50 double-spaced pages, including some 20 figures and tables. He sent me a manuscript of well over 100 pages, with some 50 or 60 figures. We reviewed his manuscript together, and he reduced it to the contracted size for my book. He subsequently used the excess prose and illustrations to create a separate authored book.

Revising Ruthlessly

There is a truism: The best works are not written; they are rewritten. Medical author Abraham Verghese advises: "Write a lot and remember that the art is in revision" [2]. For example, Ernest Hemingway rewrote the last page of *Farewell to Arms* 39 times.

Somehow it seems that inexperienced writers tend to submit their work before it has been thoroughly polished; veteran writers are more likely to submit their work to a number of revisions before tapping the "send" key dispatching the article or book chapter to an editor.

Sharing Drafts

Experienced authors field-test their work on a trusted informal critic at some time in the creative process. The ideal informal critic is objective, fearless, and not overly concerned with the artistic sensitivities of the writer. For some of the most successful writers, this has been the spouse—generally the wife. In most instances, however, the informal critic is a colleague or mentor, often not formally acknowledged in print, but an important contributor to the final publication, nonetheless.

Seeing Possibilities Others May Not See

How many physicians saw patients with tremor, bradykinesia, and rigidity before James Parkinson wrote *An Essay on The Shaking Palsy*, published in 1897? [3] (see Fig. 4.1).

Maurice Raynaud was almost certainly not the first to observe individuals with symmetrical peripheral gangrene [4]. He did however provide the first lucid description of what was to be called Raynaud disease, and he did so in 1862, the year he was awarded his doctor of medicine degree. In 1917, Leo Buerger described a condition he called presenile spontaneous gangrene; today we call this Buerger disease [5].

The point of these three examples is not that the authors mentioned have been awarded eponymous recognition. Instead, what distinguished them was that they saw what others saw, recognized its significance, and wrote about it. Louis Pasteur (see Fig. 4.2) is famous for saying, "In the fields of observation, chance favors only the prepared mind" [6].

When it comes to research, rather than recognizing the existence of previously undescribed diseases, the experienced investigator—and subsequently author—thinks of questions no one else has asked. In the 1970s, a pertinent question was the following: What are we missing in patients with the "gay bowel syndrome?" More recently, the question has been the following: What is the original source of the newly defined Middle Eastern respiratory syndrome (MERS)?

AN

ESSAY

ON THE

SHAKING PALSY.

———

BY

JAMES PARKINSON,

MEMBER OF THE ROYAL COLLEGE OF SURGEONS.

———

LONDON:

PRINTED BY WHITTINGHAM AND ROWLAND,
Goswell Street,

FOR SHERWOOD, NEELY, AND JONES,

PATERNOSTER ROW.

◆

1817.

L

Fig. 4.1 *An Essay on the Shaking Palsy* by James Parkinson, 1897 [42]

Fig. 4.2 French biologist Louis Pasteur (1822–1895) [43]

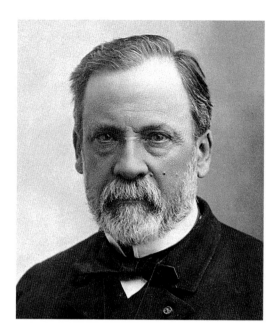

Some investigators and authors also see connections others have not described, walking conceptual paths others have not traveled. This is the essence of the book *How Doctors Think* by physician-author Jerome Groopman [7]. In this popular book, the author attempts to bridge the chasm between the fallibility of physicians and how patients can help to avoid medical misadventures.

Writing Often

If you are a professional athlete you train regularly. You need to keep muscles toned and reflexes sharp. If you are a chef, you cook daily, trying new variations of your favorite recipes. And if you are a writer, you write whenever you can. Ernest ("Papa") Hemingway wrote 500 words a day. Scottish physician author Scottish physician and author of *The Citadel,* A.J. Cronin, penned an astounding 5000 words daily, thanks to painstaking prior planning. Few of us can achieve such a level of productivity, but every serious medical writer should be composing or revising at every opportunity.

Write even if you believe you don't have time. Write something that isn't perfect—yet. Write when you think you have nothing to write about. Write a letter to your Mom. Write a poem, even if you are not a poet. Write a journal entry. Just write something to keep your mental writing "muscle" in shape.

Sometimes you just don't feel kissed by the Muse. Competing activities—watching a football game, going to the mall, eating, or sleeping—beckon seductively. Write anyhow. Some of your best work may emerge on the screen. Write a little, even if not inspired at the onset. The fourth century BCE Greek statesman and orator Demosthenes had a solution to writing inertia. He would shave one side of his head, and wouldn't leave the house until his hair again looked normal. This enforced confinement gave him time to write [8].

On the other hand, I came across a website on which a viewer asked, "What advice do you have for someone who has had writer's block for the past 6 or 7 years?" The response was, "This will sound harsh, but you're probably not a writer" [9].

What Can I Do When I Seem to Have "Writer's Block?"

There are a number of time-tested, and often effective, ways to deal with a blank screen. Get up and go for a walk. Drink more coffee. Google your topic and see what you find. Use the WIRMS (What I really mean to say) exercise: That is, try to express, out loud and in one sentence, the core message you want to get across. Here is one more suggestion.

In her essay titled "Becoming a Productive Academic Writer," Susan R. Johnson advises that you "write to think." You may not know what you really want to say until you get the first words on the screen. In doing this, try to think with your fingers, and definitely not with the editing part of your brain [10]. Yes, I know this is contrary to my exhortation to plan your writing and to outline before starting. But, we are dealing with writer's block! Desperate measures are needed. For example, when I set out to write the introduction to this chapter on "Pointers and Pitfalls," I didn't know what I was really going to say. Yes, I had a lot of notes about the eventual content: habits of the best writers, a suggestion to remedy writer's block, The Dizzy Awards, The Gunning Fog Index, coauthor issues, and the inevitable errata. I knew I had to mention the two topics in the chapter title: pointers and pitfalls. But I didn't know how I would start and finish the Introduction section. So I just began typing. What you read above is not the first draft I typed, or the second or third version. But my early effort helped generate a final iteration I could accept.

In the Introduction to This Chapter, You Mention Issues That May Arise with Coauthors: What Are Some of These?

Because authorship of published scientific articles is the ticket to academic advancement, and because science is much more complex than it was in the days of Jenner and Pasteur, today's best research is the product of shared wisdom and experience. This results in coauthorship of research reports, which introduces the human issues related to persons with diverse skills and status working together on a complicated project.

The International Committee of Medical Journal Editors (ICMJE) recommends that authorship be based on the following four criteria, which I am presenting verbatim as stated in the ICMJE website [11]:

1. Substantial contributions to the conception or design of the work, or the acquisition, analysis, or interpretation of data for the work.
2. Drafting the work or revising it critically for important intellectual content.
3. Final approval of the version to be published.
4. Agreement to be accountable for all aspects of the work in ensuring that questions related to the accuracy or integrity of any part of the work are appropriately investigated and resolved.

In addition to being accountable for the parts of the work he or she has done, an author should be able to identify which coauthors are responsible for specific other parts of the work. In addition, authors should have confidence in the integrity of the contributions of their coauthors. All those designated as authors should meet all four criteria for authorship, and all who meet the four criteria should be identified as authors [11].

The criteria for authorship described above are important, and sometimes present ethical issues when determining who will be listed as an author of a paper and in what order. But there are also some basic interpersonal issues that can complicate coauthorship, especially when it comes to preparing a report of original research.

In an ideal world, there is a captain of the ship, typically the one who generated the idea for the work and assembled the research/writing team. Then, there may be the clinician who provides access to subjects, the research methods specialist, the statistician, the acknowledged writing expert, and the acolyte who contributes hours of extra effort while learning research and writing skills. Such a team may actually function smoothly, without issues such as the following:

The Slacker

In many ways being on writing team is similar to being on a basketball or track team. Success calls for everyone to do their best and work for the good of the group. But we have all been on teams with a slacker—one who is late with data, who skips meetings, and whose actions are affecting everyone.

As soon as a slacker is identified, that person must be confronted, either by the team leader or by the whole team together. When I was at Wake Forest University School of Medicine, we called this a "prayer meeting." Following the confrontation, behavior must improve dramatically or the person must be replaced.

The Prima Donna

I was once part of a writing team; the article we were writing concerned diabetes mellitus. One of the members of the team happened to be a type 1 diabetic, and she believed that this fact accorded her primacy over all the rest of us whenever a content decision was made. There could be no questioning her decisions; after all, she had personal experience with the disease and the rest of us did not.

A blog by Bernard Lo, MD, describes a prima donna problem: "The senior author describes the second author as demanding and persistent in his opinions. Revisions have been a 'marathon' because the second author is accusatory and insulting when others do not accept his suggestions" [12]. The blog offers some potentially useful suggestions to this problem: addressing emotional issues directly, acknowledging the second author's feelings, trying to find common ground, and getting to agreement on process. If all fail, a neutral third party might be called to mediate.

The Perseverator

This person is probably a strong "P" (perceiver) in the Myers-Briggs Personality Type Indicator. A perseverator on the research team can create endless revision sessions. These begin with the first draft of a research protocol and continue through the final draft of the paper. Every noun, verb, and modifier must be debated. Eventually team members roll their eyes, throw up their hands, and allow the word-smithing perseverator to prevail, often to the detriment of the final product.

The Outlier

Sometimes just one member of a writing team has a strong opinion not shared by colleagues. And sometimes you will be the outlier. I came across one such instance on an academic website: One frustrated author writes, "I am a junior member on a research project. We have written a paper. I feel the work is not ready for publication and have issues. We have discussed the issues, and other members of the group including the lead author agree with me that there are issues. But the lead author who is more senior is too eager to get the results published, to the extent that he is ready to mislead the reviewers/readers by exaggerating and misrepresenting the partial inconclusive results to get the paper accepted. I don't think I can convince him to allow more time for the project to reach a more satisfactory stage before publication. I am rather junior and have limited say on the project. I am new to the field of the project, and the senior author is established in the field and publishes several papers in top venues each year. Other members of the project are his students" [13]. This outlier has an ethical problem, one that just might result in withdrawal from the project.

The Overlord

Let's imagine that I am one of a team of investigators in a medical school department chaired by a prestigious Nobel laureate. While the Chairman has been speaking in Paris and Buenos Aires, we have completed our study and are on the near-final draft of our paper. Suppose the department policy is that our Chairman's name be added as the terminal author on the paper. After all, the work was done in "his" laboratory. Should we agree to this? As repugnant as it may seem, having a world-famous author included on our author list may increase its chances of acceptance.

In an instance such as this, it would be time to review the ICMJE criteria for authorship, described above [11]. The peripatetic Chairman may qualify for criterion 3, blessing the final version of the paper to be submitted. But the overlord would seem to fail criteria 1, 2, and 4. Now who on the team will be chosen to tell him this?

Given the Potential Problems, Should I Ever Have One or More Coauthors?

Despite the problems that may arise with coauthors, there are times when a writing team—two or more coauthors—will produce the best work. In writing for the stage, think of Richard Rodgers and Arthur Hammerstein, who wrote productions that included "Oklahoma!" and "Carousel." Paul Simon and Art Garfunkel (Think of "Mrs. Robinson") were among my favorite songwriters and performers. We can thank the Coen brothers—Joel and Ethan—for films such as "Fargo," "Raising Arizona," and "True Grit."

Book writing coauthors include William Strauss and Neil Howe who collaborated to write *Generations,* Paul Tieger and Barbara Barron-Tieger who coauthored *Do What You Are*, and Lee and Norma Barr who wrote *The Leadership Equation.* Carole Bland and William Bergquist together wrote an analysis of mature academicians titled, *The Vitality of Senior Faculty Members: Snow on the Roof—Fire in the Furnace.* There is a book, written for medical students, titled *Making It in Medical School*, by coauthors Robert H. Coombs and Joanne St. John. Although technically coeditors rather than coauthors, Richard Reynolds and John Stone collaborated to produce a collection of stories, poems, and essays about medicine titled *On Doctoring.*

As I searched for items for the list above, I was struck by how many coauthors were married couples and how few books—medical or otherwise—have more than two coauthors.

Fischbach et al. hold that the physician and the patient are *coauthors* of the medical record [14]. The clinical record, much more than some boxes checked on a computer screen, is the patient's story, and it is the physician's job to see that it is told in the best way possible. Metaphorically, and according to Brody, when a patient is sick, his or her "story is broken," and the goal of the clinical process is to repair the story [15]. Thus, together, the patient and physician create the clinical narrative, with all the joys and perils of coauthorship.

There are other reasons to have coauthors, sometimes many of them. No multi-institutional research study will have a single author, and the reports of such studies often have a dozen or more coauthors. In addition, the editors of large multi-chapter reference books, sometimes with more than a hundred contributors, generally find that coeditors are needed. They also find that many chapter authors choose to write their chapters in concert with colleagues.

So, coauthorship can be an effort-saving decision that makes the work better than any individual could alone. Or signing on to a writing team can bring frustration and even antipathy. As with choosing a life mate, make your commitment with great care.

Does How Authors Are Listed on an Article Matter?

Yes, how you are listed among multiple authors matters. The first author is assumed, rightfully, to be the principal investigator and the person who brought the project to completion. But who comes next in the author list?

The key fact is that when a multi-author paper is cited, the custom is to list the first three authors and identify the others as "et al." Thus, in citations of the paper, only the names of the three first authors will be noted. Being a fourth or fifth author on a paper may not compromise your curriculum vitae when it comes time for promotion, but your colleagues won't see your name when others cite the work you have helped publish.

What Are Some Rookie Errors in Medical Writing?

Having selected a topic and decided on authorship, it is time to think about writing. Careful planning can help you avoid some of the common mistakes we encounter.

- *Failing to focus on the topic early in the article.* The attention span of the busy clinician can be very brief. State your thesis in the first sentence, or least the second. Consider beginning with a relevant case study, always intriguing to the professional who sees patients daily.
- *Wandering off the reservation.* This happens when you deviate from the outline and begin introducing peripheral topics. At the end of every paragraph, ask yourself if what you have just written advances your thesis and leads toward your conclusion. If adding an item "just to get it in," take it out.
- *Creating paragraphs that are too long.* Very long paragraphs leave your reader breathless. They can prompt "skipping ahead" in your article, or even abandonment to read something less tiring. One way to break up what could become an

endless paragraph is to separate the content into bullet points, as I have done with the section you are now reading.

- *Failing to provide headings.* Headings break up the text, and allow your reader a chance to breathe. Headings also create "white space" so that your writing does not appear crowded on the page.
- *Using too many adjectives and adverbs, and not enough nouns and verbs.* Nouns and verbs are strong words; descriptors are weak words. Every time you feel the urge to modify a noun, think of a phrase such as "a very large tome." In fact, part of the connotation of a *tome* is that it is "large," and that descriptor is redundant. The word "very" in the phrase is even more useless. Mark Twain advised a writer: "Substitute 'damn' every time you're inclined to write 'very;' your editor will delete it and the writing will be just as it should be" [16]. Damn good advice!
- *Introducing too many abbreviations.* Remember that not every disease you mention needs to have an abbreviation or acronym. If you mention, for example, idiopathic intracranial hypertension (IIH), and you will mention the disease only once again, on page 14 of your article manuscript, then no abbreviation is needed, although you may choose to use one. The custom is to introduce an abbreviation with first use of a term, and subsequently the term or the abbreviation can be used. But thoughtful writers refrain from creating abbreviation overload when an article discusses multiple diseases. Also keep in mind that abbreviations can be confusing. IIH, the reasonable abbreviation for idiopathic intracranial hypertension, can also be the abbreviation for idiopathic infantile hypercalcemia or iodine-induced hyperthyroidism. The abbreviation MI can stand for myocardial infarction, mental illness, and several other entities.
- *Presenting facts without citations.* Above I alluded to the patient's story being "broken" and the medical encounter as intended to "fix" the narrative. This was a concept introduced a few decades ago by physician-ethicist Howard Brody. I not only give credit to Brody for the metaphor; I also told you where you could look to find more about the concept. To present the image without attribution would have been plagiarism; to mention Brody as the author of the concept without offering a citation would have been cruel to the inquisitive reader.

What Are Some Recent Changes in the Language Used in Medical Writing Today?

Some might say we have entered an era of medical linguistic sensitivity and even political correctness. The goal seems to be to humanize the patient while removing words that connote that disease can cause pain, disability, or even death. First the patient: "Case" has become "patient." "Male" has become "man," and "female" is now woman. And we no longer refer to our patient as "the gall bladder in room 720." Well and good. We do, still, find the patient's behavior being described in accusatory terms: he "failed" chemotherapy, as if the lack of response to the latest cytotoxic drug is somehow the patient's fault.

In regard to being sick, we seem determined to minimize, even euphemize, disease, at least as far as medical writing is concerned. Patients no longer "suffer" hypertension or fracture; they are not "victims" of cancer or stroke. We even seem to have acquired an aversion to using disease as an adjective, i.e., diabetic patient or a hemophilic infant. Part of this effort is the war on traditional but now "unacceptable" disease names. Leprosy, a disease historically associated with social stigma, is now Hansen disease, contrary to the modern campaign to eliminate eponymous designations such as von Recklinghausen disease, Pott puffy tumor, and Lou Gehrig disease.

A disturbing trend is use of the generic term "provider," whether referring to a physician or anyone else with a stethoscope draped around the neck. You can go online and read the "California Department of Insurance Health Insurance Covered Lives Report," using a term "covered lives" that I find especially dehumanizing [17]. And please, let us not ever begin to refer to our patients as "clients," which has a history of describing a "lawyer's customer" [18].

Words matter. How we say things not only describes ideas and entities; it influences how we think about them.

Are There Forbidden Words in Medical Writing?

The short answer to the question "Are there forbidden words in medical writing?" is no. There are no published lists of approved and prohibited words. Of course, there are words that would offend any reasonable reader, such as racial or ethnic epithets, obvious profanity, or gratuitous slurs. No serious medical writer would use these terms. My question was in reference to "clinical" words that describe body parts and function: penis, vagina, breast, vulva, anus, and even cunnilingus and fellatio, words that might be inappropriate in some literary settings. All of these and more are found in respected medical journals. Sometimes an editor will suggest a euphemism, but there is no agreed-upon set of banned words in medical writing.

With that said, it is interesting to look at the history of written words thought to be offensive in their time. An early contributor to the problem was actually a physician named Thomas Bowdler. In the 1800s Bowdler and his sister Henrietta were apparently shocked at some of the words and deeds described in Shakespeare's plays. They removed the offending items from the Bard's works and published the results as *The Family Shakspeare* (SIC). (Note the nineteenth-century spelling of the poet's name in the title of their publication.) Pleased with their work, the Bowdlers next turned their efforts to a sanitization of *The Decline and Fall of the Roman Empire* [19]. For their dubious contribution to literature, Doctor Bowdler and Henrietta were recognized with the eponym *bowdlerize*, meaning censorship of literature to remove what is considered offensive or improper.

We have seen recent versions of Mark Twain's book *Huckleberry Finn* in which the author's word "nigger" has been replaced with "slave" throughout. In 2010, Rosa's Law was signed by President Obama, changing the classification "mentally retarded"

Fig. 4.3 John Langdon Down, who described what we now call Down syndrome [44]

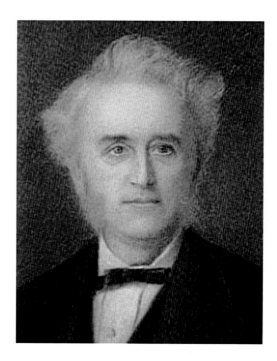

to "intellectually disabled." The law is named for 9-year-old Rosa Marcellino, who has Down syndrome and whose family championed the legislation [20].

Down syndrome, itself, has an interesting backstory of out-of-favor words. In his original description of the disease and in recognition of shared facial characteristics of affected persons, in 1866 English physician John Langdon Down used the descriptive term "mongoloid" to describe "an ethnic classification of idiots" [21] (see Fig. 4.3). The disorder came to be known as "mongolism." Citing possible misleading racial connotations of the term, a group of scientists called for a change in 1961, and in 1965, based on a request from a delegate from Mongolia, the World Health Organization (WHO) dropped the term "mongolism" [22]. Today, in contrast to the current efforts to eliminate eponymous disease names in favor of descriptive terms, we call the disorder Down syndrome. Mongolism, it seems, is actually a forbidden word.

The Associated Press has purged the terms illegal immigrant, Islamism, homophobia, and Islamophobia from its Stylebook [23]. The *Expurgated Scrabble Players Dictionary* has a long list of unacceptable words. You won't see these on a Scrabble Board: boobie, bubby, crapper, dykey, fatso, honkie, popish, redneck, squaw, and wetback [24]. On my trip to the Galapagos Islands, we saw blue-footed boobies, and why are we disrespecting the man whose name is forever linked to the flush toilet, Thomas Crapper? The *Urban Dictio*nary defines bubby as "a sweet name for someone you love." Is there something offensive about that?

As we return to medical writing and words not likely to survive editing, what we tend to find are obsolete medical terms:

- *Bright disease.* This was what we used to call glomerulonephritis or nephritis. Sorry, Richard Bright, but your name has been buried by the foes of eponyms.
- *Dementia praecox.* The original name of what we now know as schizophrenia was coined by Professor Arnold Pick to mean "premature dementia" or "premature madness."
- *Dropsy.* Derived from a Greek term meaning water, dropsy is now called edema. The older term just seems to have gone out of fashion.
- *Gay bowel syndrome.* This was a way station on our path to recognizing the human immunodeficiency virus (HIV) and the acquired immunodeficiency syndrome (AIDS).
- *Hysteria.* The Greek word *hystera* means uterus, and the world long believed that the psychiatric symptoms related to "hysteria" were somehow related to the uterus and were found only in women.
- *Melancholia.* Hippocrates believed that what we now call depression was caused by an excess of "black bile," one of the four humors of the body. Symptoms described by Hippocrates were "fear and despondencies" [25].
- *Moron.* This term was once used in psychology to describe "mild intellectual disability." As "moron" became popular as an insult, it became unpopular in the scientific literature.

To be sure I had not missed a "blacklist" somewhere, I searched the Instructions to Authors of several of my favorite medical and scientific journals for a list of forbidden words. I found none.

What Are the Dizzy Awards and Why Don't You Want to Receive One?

In the past few sections I have discussed medical writing pointers—some important ones including coauthor issues, rookie errors, and appropriate word selection. This section, describing some literary pitfalls, is presented as a humorous interlude in my otherwise serious chapter.

The Dizzy Awards, created some three decades ago, honor legendary 1930s baseball pitcher and, subsequently, sportscaster, Jay Hanna ("Dizzy") Dean who became famous for mangling the English language with expressions such as "Zarilla slud into third!" The Awards are "given for excellence in unintentionally comical, bewildering, or downright terrible medical writing"—and editing. As a sample, here are just three recent Dizzy Awards, quoted directly from the report [26]:

The Batty Title Award

Screening for Prostate Cancer in Long-Term Care
Does Long-Term Care need to bend over?

The "Who's on First?" Award

Dr. Ash had already attempted to treat the eminent patient with the usual remedies, but his condition was worsening with each passing hour.
   Sorry about Dr. Ash, but what about his patient?

The Rookie of the Year Award

He had been born in South America and emigrated to the United States several years earlier
...
   Now that's what we call a hyperactive fetus.

I recommend that each medical writer should review the latest list of Dizzy Awards as an exercise in seeing just how imprecise our prose can be, even without trying [26]. Access Reference 26 below or Google "Dizzy medical writing and editing."

What Is the Fog Index and How Can Using the Index Improve My Writing?

The Fog Index, aka the Gunning Fog Index, measures the readability of written text. It intended to indicate how easy or difficult it is for a reader to comprehend a paragraph or entire essay. Here is the calculation: Multiply the average number of words in sentences plus percentage of words with three or more syllables times 0.4. The result is the Fog Index—the number of years of education a reader needs to comprehend what you have written [27].

The website *UsingEnglish.com* describes the Fog Index of some well-known publications: *Time* magazine has a Fog Index about 11; that is, it is written at the comprehension level of a person with 11 years of education. The Fog Index for the *New York Times* is about 11–12; and professional prose, which I assume to include medical writing, "almost never exceeds 18" [27]. Just to do a little math: 12 years of school, 4 of college, and 4 of medical school is 20 years, and so medical reports should be well within the comprehension of all physicians, and most other health professionals, as well.

To test current writing, you or I can readily, but somewhat laboriously, perform the calculation described above. But there is an easier way—a (free) website that will make the reckoning for you. Just paste your paragraph into the box found at *gunning-fog-index.com*. I tested this by copying and pasting to the site the first paragraph under the question above, the sentence beginning, "The Fog Index, aka the Gunning Fog Index, measures readability ...." I quickly learned that the paragraph contained 77 words, 11 three-syllable-plus words, and 6 major punctuation marks to yield a Gunning Fog Index of 10.6 [28]. This means that at least for this paragraph of the book, a high school junior should be able to read and understand my words.

Just to see the result, I applied the Fog Index to the opening words of Sir William Osler's Aequanimitas, the valedictory address given to medical students graduating at the University of Pennsylvania, May 1, 1889 [29]:

> To many the frost of custom has made even these imposing annual ceremonies cold and lifeless. To you, at least of those present, they should have the solemnity of an ordinance — called as you are this day to a high dignity and to so weighty an office and charge.

Even allowing for somewhat formal prose of more than a century ago that seems a little stuffy today, Osler's words have a Gunning Fog Index of 14.6, well within the education level of his audience — then and now.

For those interested in this sort of determination, there are others: The Flesch-Kincaid Index describes readability by comparing the number of words in sentences to the number of syllables in words. The Lexical Density Test indicates reading difficulty or ease by the ratio of different words to the total number of words used in text. The Passive Index tells how often the writer uses passive verb forms.

For me, the Gunning Fog Index is the most useful. It is not only most understandable, telling the educational level at which the prose is comprehensible, but there is also the easy-to-use website to do your calculation.

The Fog Index Seems to Imply That Short Words Enhance Readability: Is This Really True for Medical Writing?

In writing, in general, it is axiomatic that short, strong words are best. Sir Winston Churchill, awarded the 1953 Nobel Prize in Literature, tells us: "Broadly speaking, the short words are best and the old words best of all" [30] (see Fig. 4.4). I calculated the Gunning Fog Index for this quote: 5.6. That is, this sentence should make sense to a fifth grader.

Based upon the above, I presume that if Churchill were a medical writer, he would prefer the word "gut" to "abdomen" and "leg" to "lower extremity." The use of the phrase "bilateral lower extremities" instead of "both legs" would have caused him great distress. Yet in medicine, we have an immense and complex vocabulary that includes only a few of the old, strong words. The recent edition of *Dorland's Illustrated Medical Dictionary* has 2176 pages. Most medical words found in Dorland's are patched together from prefixes, roots, and suffixes based on ancient Greek and Latin syllables to yield fairly precise terms: Think of the origins of medical words such as antimicrobial, dysdiadochokinesia, and parathyroidectomy. Thus, the specificity required for scientific reporting often necessitates the use of words that are neither short nor strong. It is better to denote "hypersomnia" than to use the phrase such as "a state in which one sleeps too much," even though this descriptive phrase has only words of one syllable.

Yet the need for precision in medical writing cannot justify unnecessary use of long, complex words (and sentences). Here is an example, cited by Fred et al., that found its way into print: "Mutations in tuberous sclerosis complex (TSC) genes are

Fig. 4.4 Statesman and author Sir Winston Churchill (1874–1965) [45]

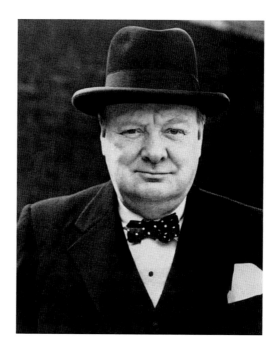

associated with dysregulated mammalian target of rapamycin (mTOR)/Akt signaling and unusual neoplasms called perivascular epithelioid cell tumors (PEComas), including angiomyolipomas (AMLs) and lymphangioleimyomatosis (LAM)" [26]. This sentence has a Gunning Fog Index of 30.3; the intended reader must be very well educated, indeed.

As a coda to the "short word" discussion, William Faulkner once criticized the writing of 1954 Nobel Prize in Literature awardee Ernest Hemingway, asserting that "he has never used a word that might send the reader to the dictionary." Hemingway responded, "Poor Faulkner. Does he really think big emotions come from big words? He thinks I don't know the ten-dollar words. I know them all right. But there are older and simpler and better words, and those are the ones I use" [31].

But in Medical Writing, Shouldn't I Strive for Erudition?

Here are two sentences from a book *about* medical writing (a book I did not write) [32]:

> The genres of medical writing have changed and new genres evolve. Genres can be considered as emerging, existing, and evolving through intertextual relationships between texts and their predecessors, as texts reproduce and also modify stylistic conventions used in texts belonging to the same genre or what comes to be recognized as such.

The second sentence above has a Gunning Fog Index of 25.81, suggesting that I need 25+ years of formal education to comprehend it on first reading. Although I am a physician, I lack this lofty educational attainment. The two sentences required me to reread them several times, and they caused my mind to wander. Is the writer referring to fairly recent innovations such as structured abstracts, or perhaps something else? The author aimed for unwarranted complexity and elegant prose at the expense of clarity.

With all the Spellchecking, Editing, and Proofreading That Go into a Medical Paper Today, Why Are Errors Still a Problem?

In a Florida shopping mall, some classical scholar, inspired by the quotation by Euripides, had these words carved in stone: "Judge a tree from it's fruit; not its leaves." Even my MS Word spellchecker picked up the error, an inappropriate apostrophe.

Benjamin Franklin once wrote: "If I were allowed to live (my life) over again, I should make no objection, only wishing for leave to do what authors do in a second edition of their works, correct some of my errata" [33]. But wouldn't it be wonderful if our lives and our writing could be error-free the first time around?

Here is a slightly embarrassing 2014 misprint. The cover of the September 24, 2014, issue of *Journal of the American Medical Association* (JAMA) contains the Table of Contents. The first research report is listed as "Effect of Enhanced Information, Effect of Enhanced Information, Values Clarification, and Removal of Financial Barriers on Use of Prenatal Genetic Testing: A Randomized Clinical Trial" (SIC). Then on page 1210 we find the full report, with a title that begins "Effect of Enhanced Information, Values Clarification, and Removal of Financial Barriers ...." The duplication of the phrase "Effect of Enhanced Information" in the Table of Contents probably causes some discomfiture to the proofreader tasked with checking the journal's cover.

Errors, and subsequent corrections, give rise to a recurring section in today's medical journals.

In Chap. 1, I told of errors of in the recently published *Diagnostic and Statistical Manual of Mental Disorders, 5th edition*. Here are correction notices describing some others:

- In the January 2009 issue of the *American Journal of Surgery* is this notation: "In the article 'Emergent embolization of the gastroduodenal artery in the treatment of upper gastrointestinal bleeding. The experience from a surgeon-initiated interventional program' by Burris JM, Lin PH, Johnston WF, Huynh TT and Kougias P. (*Am J Surg* 2009;198:59–63) the Results section of the Abstract reported in error 'The 30-day mortality rate was 8 %.' This should read 'The 30-day mortality rate was 12.5 %.'" I suspect this change could make a difference in how readers think about the procedure.

- The June 26, 2014, issue of the *New England Journal of Medicine* (NEJM) has an embarrassing correction: "Ibrutinib Resistance in Chronic Lymphocytic Leukemia. (June 12, 2014;370:2352–4). In the list of authors (page 2354), Mr. Perez's first name should have been Alexendar, rather than Alijandro." Did this author proofread the manuscript and proofs and miss the incorrect spelling of his own name? In searching the Web, I found several other corrections involving author names. Careful medical writers do not take for granted that their names are spelled correctly on title pages.
- The August 15, 2014, issue of *American Family Physician* describes an incorrect statistic: "The article 'Treatment of Alzheimer Disease' (June 15, 2011, p. 1403) incorrectly listed the disease prevalence of Alzheimer disease as one-third of Americans older than 85 years of age rather than one half in the first sentence of the abstract (p. 1403). The sentence should have read, 'Alzheimer disease is the most common form of dementia, affecting nearly one-half of all Americans older than 85 years.'" This is not good news for the 5.5 million Americans reported in the 2010 census to be aged 85 or older.

Both popular and medical literature offers us a rich treasury of humorous errata. Just for fun, here are a few:

The *Journal of the American Medical Association* has a regular feature titled "JAMA 100 Years Ago." Here is what I found in a recent column describing how newspapers mangled medical terms a century ago (JAMA. 1913;60(16):1230, author not cited): One newspaper described a patient dying of "pleurisy of the brain," after becoming ill "with pulmonary peritonitis." Another reporter told of a man who "while cranking his automobile sustained what is technically knows as a Colles fracture of the right rib." And another newspaper told its readers, "The bacillus *Welchii* is the gas bacillus dwelling in the international track" [34].

In his article "The Trouble with Medical Journals," Smith, former editor of the British Medical Journal, gives us a few more comical errata examples. "Corrigendum to 111th report of the Aeronautical Research Council, page 1, 4th line from the bottom of the page, delete possible and insert impossible." And, in typically elegant British style, "Due to an error in the preparation of this week's Gazette two photographs were transposed. We apologize to Councillor Ray … for suggesting he was a vegetable and to allotment owner Mr. Bernard …, whose prize-winning carrot did not make a speech at Faraday School prize giving" [35].

We also find errors in books: The first sentence of the Beverly Sills 1976 autobiography describes the author's childhood: "When I was only three, and still named Belle Miriam Silverman, I sang my first aria in pubic." If you find a copy of *God's Gold* by Bernard Malamud and read the dust jacket carefully, you find that Malamud is credited with also writing *The Centaur*. Sorry, John Updike authored that book [36].

Medical books are not exempt from errors. The *First Aid for the USMLE* review book series maintains an errata website (http://www.firstaidteam.com/updates-and-corrections) and offers a $20 Amazon gift card to anyone who identifies and reports an error. There is a special website (http://web.itu.edu.tr/cilesiz/courses/BYM501E/ Medical_instrumentation_4e_errata4.p) for Errata for the book J.G. Webster (ed.), *Medical Instrumentation: Application And Design*, 4th ed., Hoboken NJ.

An author's nightmare is a series of reader reviews citing numerous errors, as occurred in the majority of 19 reviews of *Lange Q&A Surgery, 5th edition*, as of August 23, 2014 [37]. The authors might not die of a misprint, but could succumb to embarrassment.

What Makes a Good Title for an Article or Book?

If you are like most of us opening a medical journal, you look first at the title. Then you decide if you will thumb to the paper and read the abstract. Finally, if the abstract is compelling and the topic is important to you, you may actually read the entire article, statistical analysis, and all. For books, title selection may be even important, as readers may not have an abstract or synopsis of your book to peruse.

The success of a published scientific paper is measured by the times it is cited. With current digital capabilities, this is now readily measurable. Huggett reports on a series of papers studying the various characteristics of titles of papers published in the journal *Cell* and other publications [38]. Here are some of the findings:

Length of Title

According to the report, there seemed to be no difference between short and long titles in the number of citations an article receives, but when data were subjected to statistical analysis, it turned out that the articles most cited had titles with 31–40 characters. The finding by Huggett is not consistent with the findings of a study by Habibzadeh, described in Chap. 7, showing higher citation rates for articles with longer titles [39].

Punctuation

There were more citations for papers with titles containing colons and commas, and less citations when the title contained a question mark. Only one paper studied had an exclamation mark in its title, and thus the jury is still out for that choice of punctuation. One investigator cited by Huggett, Professor Ben Blencowe, reported, "For research articles, I try to use titles that are concise while conveying the most interesting and surprising new results from the study. For review titles, I generally start with the main overall subject followed by a colon and then one or more subtopics that best describe the contents of the review" [38].

As a reader, I also prefer when the authors of a research report tell me what they found right in the title, and don't tease me with riddles or question marks. This was corroborated by a study of 423 research articles from Public Library of Science (PLoS) journals and from 12 Biomed Central (BMC) journals. The authors report: "Articles with results-describing titles were cited more often than those with methods-describing titles." This study also showed that articles with short titles are cited more often [38].

In the series reported by Huggett, the top ten papers, measured by citations, had no punctuation in their titles [38].

Humor

At least in two psychology journals studied, the Huggett report tells that articles with highly amusing titles received fewer citations [40].

In the end, the paper must pass peer review and be published before it can be cited. That calls for good-quality research and medical writing; if your paper is lacking in one or both of these characteristics, a brilliant title cannot save you.

How Do You Know When You Are Done Writing an Article or Book Chapter?

Before thinking about being finished with an article or book, you must do two things: Proofread relentlessly including checking your headings and engaging your spellchecker. Then, give the work a cooling-off period and put it away for a while. In the meantime, do something else, anything but perseverating about the work now resting on your computer. Take a short vacation, read a novel, and plan your next project. Do anything but think about the paper or book.

Then, when you almost cannot remember the exact title of the work, proofread it one more time. Then you just may be finished.

Here again is where your personality type may come into play. In Chap. 1, I described the Myers Briggs personality types. When it comes to finishing a writing project, the preference as to how you live your life exerts its influence: The perceiver (the "P") will feel the urge to continue wordsmithing and revising, and will be reluctant to let the project go on to a publisher. The judger (the "J"), on the other hand, will be anxious to declare the work *done*, and may, in fact, submit the article for review before it is really ready.

In the end, in the words of American author Thomas Farber, "A writer is someone who finishes" [41]. *War And Peace*, by Leo Tolstoy, is a three-volume, 1,400+ page epic work. At some time, Tolstoy just had to say, "It's finished."

Then it is time to get your work in print.

References

1. Author Information. Am J Cardiol. http://www.ajconline.org/authorinfo#idp1423952/.
2. Lightbourn A. Physician/writer scores big with his epic first novel. Rancho Santa Fe Rev. http://www.ranchosantafereview.com/2011/04/27/physicianwriter-scores-big-with-his-epic-first-novel/.
3. Parkinson J. An essay on the shaking palsy. London: Sherwood, Neely, and Jones; 1897.
4. Raynaud M. On local asphyxia and symmetrical gangrene of the extremities. Paris: PhD Thesis; 1862.
5. Buerger L. Thromboangiitis obliterans: a study of the vascular lesions leading to presenile spontaneous gangrene. Am J Med Sci. 1917;154:319.
6. Pasteur L. Lecture at the University of Lille, France. 7 Dec 1854.
7. Groopman J. How doctors think. New York: Houghton Mifflin; 2007.
8. Jonsson S. The 9 weirdest habits of highly effective authors. Barnes & Noble Book Blog. http://www.barnesandnoble.com/blog/the-9-weirdest-writing-habits-of-highly-effective-authors/.
9. Bendis!. http://brianmichaelbendis.tumblr.com/post/70724241561/what-advice-do-you-have-for-someone-that-has-had/.
10. Johnson SR. Becoming a productive academic writer. http://www.thrivingamidstchaos.com/files/Becoming-a-productive-academic-writer.pdf/.
11. Defining the role of authors and contributors. Int Comm Med J Eds. http://www.icmje.org/recommendations/browse/roles-and-responsibilities/defining-the-role-of-authors-and-contributors.html/.
12. Lo B. When authorship turns sour. CTST Blogs. http://accelerate.ucsf.edu/blogs/ethics/when-authorship-turns-sour/.
13. What to do when co-authors want to submit manuscript for publication and you think it still has problems? http://academia.stackexchange.com/questions/20942/what-to-do-when-co-authors-want-to-submit-manuscript-for-publication-and-you-thi/.
14. Fischbach RL et al. The patient and practitioner as co-authors of the medical record. Patient Couns Health Educ. 1980; 1st quarter, 2:1.
15. Brody H. My story is broken; can you help me fix it? Medical ethics and the joint construction of narrative. Med Lit. 1980;13:79.
16. Norquist R. Mark Twain's top ten writing tips. About education. http://grammar.about.com/od/advicefromthepros/a/TwainTips.htm/.
17. California Department of Insurance Health Insurance Covered Lives Report. http://www.insurance.ca.gov/0100-consumers/0020-health-related/coveredlivesrpt.cfm/.
18. Online Etymology Dictionary. http://www.etymonline.com/index.php?term=client.
19. Thomas Bowdler. Encyclopedia Brittanica. http://www.britannica.com/EBchecked/topic/76108/Thomas-Bowdler.
20. Thomas JE. Rosa's law changed words – now let's change prejudice. Teaching Tolerance. http://www.tolerance.org/blog/rosa-s-law-changed-words-now-let-s-change-prejudice.
21. Down JLH. Observations on an ethnic classification of idiots. London Hosp Rep. 1866;3:259.
22. Howard-Jones N. On the diagnostic term "Down's disease". Med Hist. 1979;23:102.
23. The AP Stylebook's silent killing of the term "homophobia". http://www.examiner.com/article/the-ap-stylebook-s-silent-killing-of-the-term-homophobia.
24. Words removed in The Expurgated Scrabble Players Dictionary, a.k.a. OSPD3. http://home.teleport.com/~stevena/scrabble/expurg.html.
25. Hippocrates. Aphorisms. 6:23.
26. Fred HL, et al. Dizzy medical writing and editing. Tex Heart J. 2010;37:505. http://www.ncbi.nlm.nih.gov/pmc/articles/PMC2953220.
27. Fog Index: UsingEnglish.com. http://www.usingenglish.com/glossary/fog-index.html.
28. Gunning Fog Index. http://gunning-fog-index.com.
29. Osler W. Aequanimitas and other addresses. 3rd ed. Philadelphia: Blakiston; 1932. p. 3.

30. Churchill W. Words that work. New York: Hyperion; 2007, p. 1.
31. Rovit E, et al. Hemingway and Faulkner in their time. New York: Bloombury Academic; 2006.
32. Vihla M. Medical writing: modality in focus. Amsterdam: Rodopi; 1999.
33. Benjamin Franklin. Quoted in: Isaacson W. Benjamin Franklin. New York: Simon & Schuster; 2003, p 462.
34. Reiling J, editor. JAMA 100 years ago. JAMA. 2013;309:1565.
35. Smith RS. The trouble with medical journals. Medico-Legal J. 2008;76:79.
36. McDowell E. Publishers battle the goof and the glitch. The New York Times. p C10.
37. Customer Reviews: Lange Q&A Surgery paperback, 5th ed. http://www.amazon.com/Lange-amp-Surgery-Fifth-Edition/product-reviews/0071475664/ref=cm_cr_pr_btm_link_2?ie=UTF8&pageNumber=2&showViewpoints=0&sortBy=bySubmissionDateDescending.
38. Paiva CE, et al. Articles with short titles describing the results are cited more often. Clinics (Sao Paulo). 2012;67(5):509.
39. Habibzadeh F, et al. Are shorter article titles more attractive for citations? Cross-sectional study of 22 scientific journals. Croat Med J. 2010;51:165.
40. Huggett S. Heading for success: or how not to title your paper. Res Trends. http://www.researchtrends.com/issue24-september-2011/heading-for-success-or-how-not-to-title-your-paper/.
41. Farber T. Quoted in: Hallinan T. Finishing your novel. http://www.timothyhallinan.com/writers.php.
42. Parkinson, An Essay on the Shaking Palsy (title page). Public domain. http://commons.wikimedia.org/wiki/File:Parkinson,_An_Essay_on_the_Shaking_Palsy_(title_page).png.
43. Louis Pasteur. Public domain. http://commons.wikimedia.org/wiki/File:Louis_Pasteur.jpg.
44. JLHdown. John Langdon Down. Public domain. http://commons.wikimedia.org/wiki/File:JLHdown.jpg.
45. Churchill HU 90973. Winston Churchill. This artistic work created by the United Kingdom Government is in the public domain. http://commons.wikimedia.org/wiki/File:Churchill_HU_90973.jpg.

Chapter 5
Getting Your Work in Print

You aren't really a writer until your words appear in print and you can show them to your friends and family: "Look what I wrote!" (Actually, don't be too disappointed if not all your kin share your level of excitement.) Articles, chapter, and books still hidden in computer files are just unfulfilled dreams. It is publication that makes your work "real" for you, your admirers, and the world.

This chapter is about how to get your work from your computer to some sort of publication—digital, print, or something else. The first step, for both articles and books, is the review process, an inevitable speed bump on the road to publication, with its arcane pathways, hidden biases, and occasional unfairness. There are classic reasons for rejection, which I will tell you about, and a few you may learn about for the first time. This chapter also presents some little known facts about the medical journals we all trust, and I will alert you to the opportunities and the perils of open-access publishing.

So, hang on for a rapid journey through the world of medical publishing.

What Do I Need to Know About Medical Journals and the Peer Review Process?

The number of scholarly journals grows by 3.5 % yearly, publishing some 1.8 million scholarly articles annually. As an example of the volume of activity involved, the *New England Journal of Medicine* (NEJM) receives 5000 manuscript submissions yearly and has a stable of 10,000 peer reviewers worldwide. And now we have open-access online journals, and the definition of "journal" and "publishing" is becoming murky [1].

What virtually all medical, scientific, and technology journals have in common is the peer review process, initiated in 1665 by the first editor of the *Philosophical*

© Springer International Publishing Switzerland 2015
R.B. Taylor, *What Every Medical Writer Needs to Know*,
DOI 10.1007/978-3-319-20264-8_5

Transactions of the Royal Society of London, Henry Oldenburg. Since that time, an estimated 50 million journal articles have been published [2]. Professor Larry Wasserman describes peer review as follows: "It is a centralized, secretive system that allocates scarce resources (reviewers' time) by fiat." Think of all the scholarly effort that has gone into reviewing 50 million journal articles over the years. And that number only counts the ones published, and does not include the many articles reviewed multiple times for different journals, and those reviewed and rejected, never to see print at all. He calls for scrapping the current prepublication peer review system in favor of post-publication open review, with reviewers taking ownership for their comments. But until that time comes, the following describes what today's author encounters once managing to have a paper accepted for review [3].

The editor, or some trusted minion, scans your paper for suitability for the journal. A paper on a novel approach to the management of preeclampsia of pregnancy submitted to the *American Journal of Orthopedics*, as an extreme example, would be promptly rejected without being sent out for review. If this paper on preeclampsia were, however, submitted to the *American Journal of Obstetrics & Gynecology*, and if the research methods seem to be reasonably sound, the conclusions apparently unbiased, and the paper had only a few errors of grammar and syntax, it would probably be sent out for peer review.

Peer reviewers are physicians and scientists who have some knowledge of the general field covered in the paper. Your paper will, in most instances, be "blinded," meaning that items in the manuscript that could identify the authors and their institutions have been redacted. Authors are also blinded in being unaware of who reviews their papers.

Peer reviewers are expected to read the paper critically and without bias, and then prepare a report for the editor, usually with some comment about the suitability of the paper for publication, with or without revisions. Peer reviewers receive no pay, leading to Professor Wasserman's comment about "scarce resources." If asked why they do such time-consuming work without remuneration, a peer reviewer will probably describe the imperative to give back to a system that allows his or her own papers to be reviewed.

Most papers are critiqued by three peer reviewers; this prevents the situation of one favoring publication and one reviewer recommending summary rejection. With three reviewers, there is always a majority opinion, which makes the journal editor's job easier.

The merits of the peer review process have been questioned by some, including the former editor of the *British Medical Journal* (BMJ), Richard Smith [4]:

> Medical journals, which many imagine to be as dull as telephone directories and twice as obscure, influence the lives of everybody—and not always for the better. Not only do they affect how doctors treat patients and the actions taken by public health authorities, they also influence how we think about birth, death, pain, and sickness. It may therefore make sense for you—the thoughtful but not necessarily expert reader—to pay attention to the ways of medical journals, particularly as many of those ways are deficient and need reform.

Several facts presented in this chapter call into question the objectivity and fairness of the peer review process and, in fact, the editorial decisions that follow initial peer review.

Is the Manuscript Review Process at Journals Truly Blinded?

Yes—sometimes it is. But often it is not. I have reviewed articles for a number of medical journals. Sometimes I have found the authors' names and institutions redacted, in an effort to allow a blinded review. But even then, consider that journal editors try to send papers to reviewers who are knowledgeable in the field. This means that a reviewer evaluating a paper on, for example, a new approach to hip replacement surgery will often recognize the surgical technique described or other content of the paper, and, hence without actually trying, will deduce the identity of the authors.

When Submitting a Paper for Publication, Does the Name of My Institution Matter?

I wish I could say "No," but this is not necessarily the case. There is a classic example of what sometimes happens. An eye-opening article all medical writers should read was published in 1982 in *Behavioral and Brain Sciences*. Authors Peters and Ceci [5] wondered about the adequacy and fairness of peer review practices. Here is what they did: The authors selected 12 articles by researchers in highly respected US psychology departments like Yale and Harvard. Each of these articles had been published in a different, prestigious American psychology journal with high rejection rates (80 % or greater) and non-blinded peer reviewers. Peters and Ceci substituted fictitious author names and institutions (something like the Mountain View Center for Human Potential) for the elite institution names that had been listed on the original papers. The manuscripts, with only author names and institutions changed, were then retyped and formally resubmitted to the same journals that had peer reviewed and published them 18–32 months earlier.

What happened to the 12 papers? Thirty-eight editors and reviewers evaluated the altered articles; only three papers were detected as ruses. Nine of the 12 articles were earnestly peer reviewed, resulting in an editorial decision. In the end, eight of the nine were rejected. Sixteen of 18 referees had recommended against publication. In many cases, the referees described "serious methodological flaws." In the end, authors Peters and Ceci ponder the possibility "that systematic bias was operating to produce the discrepant reviews. The most obvious candidates as sources of bias in this case would be the authors' status and institutional affiliation." And would you be surprised to learn that Peters and Ceci suffered rejection of their report by a number of journals before achieving publication?

If I Receive National Institutes of Health Support for My Research, What Are the Implications for the Published Report?

Investigators who receive National Institutes of Health (NIH) support for their research or support from NIH-funded academic medical centers are required to send their published reports to the PubMed Central public access repository. The policy applies to any manuscript that:

- Is peer reviewed.
- And is accepted for publication in a journal on or after April 7, 2008.
- And arises from:

  - Any direct funding from an NIH grant or cooperative agreement active in Fiscal Year 2008 or beyond, or
  - Any direct funding from an NIH contract signed on or after April 7, 2008, or
  - Any direct funding from the NIH Intramural Program, or
  - An NIH employee [6].

As one who spends a lot of time doing research online, I am always pleased when the article I need is in the public domain.

Berner cautions that compliance with the NIH policy is less than 100 %. Some researchers are unaware of the relatively new policy or are unaware that co-investigators are NIH supported [7].

Do Reviewers Ever Experience "Scholarly Advantage" from Information Learned During the Peer Review Process?

Certainly peer reviewers get a preview of things to come in their field. Do they ever benefit somehow from this information? Peer reviewers learn first about emerging concepts and technology in fields where the first to publish gets the credit—and often achieve success in the next round of grant funding awards. Irwin et al. report, "Not surprisingly, NIH study section members have always enjoyed a higher success rate with their own applications than the general scientific community has, with a current funding rate more than eight percent higher than the general success rate" [8]. In the grant-funding tournament that investigators rely on for ongoing support, 8 % is an advantage even a Las Vegas casino would envy.

Ethical issues can arise when the journal reviewer is sent a paper describing a study that is similar to his or her own work or that may overlap with work in progress or in the planning stages, especially if future grant-funding competition may become an issue. This reviewer should decline to review the paper and return it to the editor with an explanation. But, of course, before declining to review the paper, the reviewer has already *read* it. Academia can be a fiercely competitive arena, and the adage that "knowledge is power" applies in the world of funded research.

What Other Biases or Conflicts of Interest Might Peer Reviewers Have?

There are many possible biases a peer reviewer might hold. Let us assume that the reviewer has deduced the identity of the author(s). Suppose the reviewer and the author had a serious personal disagreement recently. Perhaps the reviewer left the author's institution under unhappy circumstances. Or on the other side of the coin, perhaps the author was your former colleague or mentor. Might that be reflected as a positive bias in your review? [9].

A strong religious belief might constitute a bias if reviewing a paper describing a technique to induce abortion. Or the reviewer and author may hold conflicting opinions on current issues in the use of stem cells.

Financial conflicts of interest can occur when papers under consideration involve commercial products, such as drugs or devices. Might the reviewer have served as a past consultant to the company sponsoring the research? If the reviewer owns a few hundred shares of Pfizer stock, does this involve a conflict of interest if reviewing a paper involving a Pfizer product?

I Am Planning to Write or Edit a Book: Are Book Proposals Also Peer Reviewed?

The best publishers of medical and scientific books send proposals for review. The process is similar to that described above for journal articles, but is just not as rigidly prescribed.

Book publishers are in the business of selling books and making money. For this reason, they are interested not only in the scientific merits of the proposed book. They also need to predict how many copies of the final volume might be sold. With this in mind, the publisher's acquisitions editor (the person who seeks out authors with good ideas for books) will scan all proposals. As with papers submitted to scholarly journals, some book proposals will be promptly rejected. A common reason stated is, "The proposed book does not meet our publishing needs at this time."

If your proposal passes initial muster with the acquisitions editor, it will probably be sent for review to scholars working in your field. In contrast to journals, the book editor may consult only one trusted reviewer. Questions the publisher might ask the reviewer to consider include the following [10]:

- What is your opinion of the overall quality of the proposed book?
- Does the book content seem to be organized rationally?
- What do you think is the audience for this book?
- Might this book be appropriate as a course text?
- How could this book, as proposed, be improved?
- Would you recommend that a contract be offered for this book?

The reviewer(s) will write an evaluation for the acquisitions editor who, before an ultimate publish-or-not decision is made, may share the review report(s) with the rest of the editorial team, who will make a joint decision about your book proposal.

Is There Somewhere I Can Find the Acceptance Rates for Various Journals?

The acceptance rate is the number of submissions that ultimately end up as printed articles, expressed as a percentage of the total submissions. The rejection rate is the acceptance rate subtracted from 100 %. For example, the *Journal of the American Medical Association* (JAMA) lists an overall acceptance rate of 9.5 % and, for research reports, the rate is 3.7 % [11]. I searched diligently but could not find any website or other list that provides a centralized comparison of journal acceptance rates. Nevertheless, knowing a journal's acceptance rate is very useful in deciding on the initial target article for your paper.

Acceptance rates for journals vary for several reasons. For instance, I believe that many papers are first submitted to the *New England Journal of Medicine* or some other prestigious journal for a free critique, even though the chances of the paper being published in that journal are slim. The ethics of this practice, which strains the resources of the journal, is open to question, but it is done, nevertheless. This sort of "free advice" practice of submitting papers doomed to rejection leads to a low acceptance rate. Another factoid: A specialty journal focusing on one disease or organ, such as *Diabetes, Hypertension,* or *Pancreas,* will generally have a higher acceptance rate than a broad-based medical journal, such as the NEMJ or BMJ, because the more general journal attracts many more submissions, some of uneven quality, than the specialized journals.

Finding and assessing acceptance rates can also be confounded by how the denominator is defined. Some journals count submissions as all papers that arrive on the journal's Submission online site; other journals may consider a paper a submission only if it is sent for peer review. Some journals simply do not maintain acceptance or rejection rates at all.

I have found what may be a useful way to find acceptance rates in your field. Search Google using "acceptance rate and (list your specialty or field of research)." Using this method, I found that, as examples, the *Journal of Clinical Psychiatry* has an acceptance rate of 28 %, *Pediatrics* lists its acceptance rate as approximately 10 %, and the *British Journal of Surgery* has a 13–19 % acceptance rate. Using the Google search method described here, I could not readily find acceptance rates for the journals *Hypertension* and *Pancreas.*

A journal's acceptance rate may be listed on the official website, or not. The website of *Hypertension* lists an acceptance rate of 26 %. I could not find an acceptance rate on the website of *Pancreas,* but I did learn that the journal has an impact factor of 2.953 (see Chap. 3 for a description of the impact factor). Ingersoll et al. report that, in general, the mean acceptance rates for journals that publish manuscripts in the HIV/AIDS behavioral science realm have a mean acceptance rate of 39 % [12].

If all the above fails and you are keen to know a specific journal's acceptance rate, you could send an e-mail to the journal editor's office.

What Actually Gets Published in Medical Journals? Are Peer-Reviewed Journals Unbiased in What Is Published?

According to a 2012 report in the *Washington Post*, "Over a year-long period ending in August, NEJM published 73 articles on original studies of new drugs, encompassing drugs approved by the FDA since 2000 and experimental drugs".

Of those articles, 60 were funded by a pharmaceutical company, 50 were co-written by drug company employees, and 37 had a lead author, typically an academic, who had previously accepted outside compensation from the sponsoring drug company in the form of consultant pay, grants, or speaker fees. "The *New England Journal of Medicine* is not alone in featuring research sponsored in large part by drug companies — it has become a common practice that reflects the growing role of industry money in research" [13].

As I write this, I have in front of me two issues of the *New England Journal of Medicine*. The July 17, 2014, issue (2014; 371:3) has four original articles, all about drugs and all at least partially supported by pharmaceutical companies. To provide some balance, the August 14, 2014, issue (2014;371:7) of the journal has three original articles about salt and one about high-dose versus standard-dose influenza vaccine. One of the salt studies was supported by the Bill and Melinda Gates Foundation, which I consider free of commercial bias. The other two studies reported "major contributions" from pharmaceutical companies. Sanofi Pasteur supported the influenza vaccine study.

Why are so many of the articles in our best journals funded by pharmaceutical companies? One reason is that private pharmaceutical funding can buy the best quality research. Struggling assistant professors with teaching responsibilities funded by small government grants just can't compete with Sanofi Pasteur. And when the research is completed, pharmaceutical companies have the funds to hire professional writers to prepare the paper for publication.

As if pharmaceutical research studies did not have enough advantage in the publication sweepstakes, in an article in *American Scholar*, Washington writes: "Moreover, drug makers sometimes agree to buy journal advertising only if it is accompanied by favorable editorial mentions of their products. Or their in-house stables of writers or hired pens generate 'advertorials,' a Frankensteinian mix of medical content and marketing messages that can be indistinguishable from editorial material." Washington also quotes Richard Smith: "Pharmaceutical firms also inform journals," Smith observes, "that they are receptive to buying huge volumes of reprints that favor their wares: The profits for the journal can easily reach $100,000" [14].

Part of the journal editor's job description is to help assure that the publication is profitable. If choosing to publish a paper on a lifestyle health issue such as smoking or overeating versus a drug-related paper with the promise of the purchase of a huge number of reprints, which might the editor select?

In view of the above, is it any wonder that according to Kesselheim et al. the fact that a research study has industry sponsorship negatively influences physicians' opinion of the quality of the research and reduces willingness to put the results into practice, even if the study was properly conducted. The authors suggest, "These effects may influence the translation of clinical research into practice" [15].

How Quickly Is My Article Likely to Be Published After Completion of the Study?

You have completed your landmark research study on reduction in the size of kidney stones by daily consumption of broccoli. How long will it be before you see it in print? The answer is: probably quite a while. Two recently published studies document the delay. Ross et al. reviewed 1336 clinical trials published during calendar year 2009; they found that the median time from completion of the study to publication was 21 months [16]. Gordon et al. studied 244 randomized clinical trials funded by the National Heart, Lung, and Blood Institute completed during calendar years 2000–2011; they reported that less than two-thirds were in print within 30 months of completion of the study [17]. Note that these times begin with completion of the study, not with acceptance of the paper by the journal.

Why so long? When the study is completed, the writing begins. This often takes months, longer if there develops a clash of egos among the research team or if one of the groups is a compulsive rewriter and persnickety wordsmither.

Then, after initial acceptance by the journal, there are the inevitable revisions needed in response to reviewer and editorial suggestions. Often there are several rounds of such changes. Then, of course, after all authors, reviewers, and editors are in accord, there are the "typesetting" and the proofreading stages.

Yes, getting from completed study to printed page takes a long time. The process has a lot of steps, and not all problems lie with the journals. Authors must shoulder the responsibility for some of the delays.

How Quickly Will My Paper Be Published After It Has Been Accepted by a Journal?

Against all odds, your paper has been accepted for publication in a respected medical journal. How long before you see in print? Sometimes you can find publication timelines on the journal's website. For example the *Journal of the American Medical Association* website describes [18]:

- Time to first decision overall: 3 days for initial decision without review; 40 days with review.

- Fast publication: 2–22 days for Online First publication and 35 days for publication in print.

I searched the websites of the *Journal of Emergency Medicine* and *Pediatrics* for similar information about time to first decision and time to publication. I learned about journals' circulation and impact factor, but could not find the time-to-publication data I was looking for.

On the other hand, a Google search of "time to publication" followed by the name of the journal will sometimes give you the information you seek. For example, by this method I learned that the journal *Gut* has an average time between acceptance and final publication (on line) of 19 days [19]. Note that the time to online publication will almost certainly be much shorter than the time from acceptance to publication for articles appearing in print.

If you really need to know the time intervals between submission and a decision or between a decision and publication, an e-mail to the journal's editorial office may give you the information you seek.

What Should I Know About Open-Access Publications?

How many times have you or I searched for the results of a study important to the work you are doing and encountered a journal's website requiring a subscription or at least a 1-day payment for the privilege of viewing the full research report?

Open-access publication offers an alternative to this frustration.

With a mantra attributed to futurist Stewart Brand, "Information wants to be free," the advocates of open-access publishing see their online journals as the logical extension of the transition of most print journals adapting online platforms over the past two decades [20]. Of course, *free* can mean "liberated," and it can also mean "without cost." Sometimes you have to pick one.

The poster child for open-access publishing is *PLOS ONE*, which in 2013 published its 100,000th manuscript, making it now the largest journal in the world [21]. A peer-reviewed open-access journal published online by the Public Library of Science (PLOS), *PLOS ONE* began in 2006 as a weekly publication and is now published daily. The journal espouses a philosophy of "publish first, judge later." There is, however, prepublication review of submissions. Following publication, an article is subject to comments, rating, and online annotation by viewers.

PLOS ONE has been awarded the *Publishing Innovation Award* presented by the Association for Learned and Professional Society Publishers. Researchers who are concerned about a journal's impact factor will be relieved to learn that the *PLOS ONE* impact factor for 2013 was a respectable 3.535 [22]. For comparison, the 5-year impact factor for the journal *Academic Medicine* is 3.076 and for the *Journal of General Internal Medicine* is 3.646.

PLOS ONE is actually the flagship of a fleet of seven journals, including *PLOS Biology*, *PLOS Medicine*, and *PLOS Genetics*. As discussed below, there are issues in regard to open-access publishing concerning how these enterprises are funded.

There are a host of copyright issues. And there are concerns about the high acceptance rates and low rejection rates affecting the quality of publications in these online-only publications [23]. Nevertheless, the open-access journal model, pioneered by PLOS, seems to offer a view to the future.

With no pharmaceutical advertising, subscription fees, and lucrative reprints, how can *PLOS ONE* stay in business? In fact, information sharing is not "free," and PLOS pays its way by charging authors a publication fee, which can be waived if the author lacks sufficient funds. The current publication fee charged to authors by *PLOS ONE* is $1350 per article, and is more for the other six PLOS journals. The fee may be paid by the author's institution, or waived upon special request. The PLOS family has inspired an increasingly large flock of imitators, some very legitimate and some not so. With the advent of publication fees paid by authors, the potential for exploitation arises, as I will discuss next.

What Do I Need to Know About Predatory Publishers?

"Predatory publishers" are those that prey on the ambitious but naïve academician desperate to build a curriculum vitae (CV). After all, these underpaid and underappreciated assistant professors might reason, an entry on a CV is better than nothing, even if it is in a journal of questionable credibility. Scholarly communications librarian at the University of Colorado-Denver, Jeffrey Beall, coined the term "predatory publishers" [24]. These publishers all subscribe to the "gold" (i.e., author pays) open-access model.

As a professor at two medical schools and as a published author, a few years ago I began receiving e-mails inviting me to contribute articles to medical journals whose names were not familiar to me. The curious thing was that the journals usually had nothing to do with my clinical practice or my prior writings. Why would a journal ask me, a family physician, to submit a paper on brain imaging or management of an uncommon blood disorder? I even have had a few invitations to list my name as being on the editorial boards of virtually unknown scientific publications. My latest unsolicited invitation was from the *Landmark Research Journal of Management and Economics*, a curious offer because I have never written about "management and economics." Before long, and without submitting a single manuscript or joining a questionable editorial board, I deduced that I was being approached by predatory journals and publishers.

What are the lure and tactics of the predator publishers? By mining lists of academicians whose articles appear in scholarly publications, they solicit contributions to their online open-access journals, promising peer review and a chance (in fact, a very good chance) for publication. For those who take the bait, peer review may be a glance by the editor, who is often based in some distant land. Publication is highly likely; only the most flagrantly worthless papers are rejected.

The catch is the fee. All predatory journals charge a review fee or a publication fee, which is how the journal makes money. In effect, a predatory journal is an online vanity press. Its chief goal is profit.

The following is a story to show the extent of the problem. What I am about to describe is so outrageous that I advise you to read the article in its entirety [25]. Here is what happened: John Bohannon, Harvard University science journalist, wrote a paper the described astounding anticancer properties found in a compound extracted from a lichen—the green stuff that grows on wet rocks. In the author's words, "Any reviewer with more than a high-school knowledge of chemistry and the ability to understand a basic data plot should have spotted the paper's short-comings immediately. Its experiments are so hopelessly flawed that the results are meaningless." Using a fictitious name and reporting faculty status at a nonexistent institute of medicine in the city of Asmara in Eritrea (Africa), Bohannon then sub-mitted the paper, with slight modifications, to 304 open-access journals. The outra-geously faulty paper was accepted for publication by more than half of the journals. To its credit, PLOS ONE was among the journals to reject the bogus report.

Even reputable publishers can be guilty of lax reviews in their open-access journals. Again in Bohannon's words (to be sure it is said correctly) [25]:

> In 2012, Sage was named the Independent Publishers Guild Academic and Professional Publisher of the Year. The Sage publication that accepted my bogus paper is the *Journal of International Medical Research*. Without asking for any changes to the paper's scientific content, the journal sent an acceptance letter and an invoice for $3100.

There are more than a handful of perpetrators. Jeffrey Beale posts a list of preda-tory publishers, updated annually. In 2014, the list contained the names of 477 ques-tionable publishers, up from 225 in the year 2013, plus a second list of 303 questionable stand-alone journals [26].

A few years ago, Dr. Drummond Rennie, Deputy Editor of JAMA, was quoted as saying [27]:

> There seems to be no study too fragmented, no hypothesis too trivial, no literature citation too biased or too egotistical, no design too warped, no methodology too bungled, no presen-tation of results too inaccurate, too obscure, and too contradictory, no analysis too self serving, no argument too circular, no conclusions too trifling or too unjustified, and no grammar or syntax too offensive for a paper to end up in print.

We now know the home for the pitiful papers Dr. Rennie describes. It is the predatory medical journal.

The message for the astute medical writer is this: If solicited to submit a paper to a journal whose name you have never heard, delete the message. Or if curious and just a little tempted, consult Jeffrey Beale's list of predatory publishers [26]. And perhaps reread the tale of John Bohannon's sting [25].

What About Fees Paid by Authors for Rapid Review?

Medical writers submitting scholarly articles to journals will sometimes encounter the opportunity to pay for a quicker review. For example the journal *Postgraduate Medicine* levies no charge for Standard Track review, which "provides manuscript submission to online publication within 30–45 weeks." But perhaps your paper contains rapidly changing information and 45 weeks seems much too long to wait for publication. The journal has an Expedited Track which "offers submission to publication in 10–12 weeks," for a mere cost of $500 per printed page. But if your findings are red-hot and likely to be picked up by the *New York Times*, you may want the journal's Super-Fast Track promising "the top level of service–with 72-h peer review turnaround, DOI assignment upon approval of page proofs and manuscript submission to publication in 5–7 weeks." The cost for the Super-Fast Track is $750 per printed page [28]. Postgraduate Medicine has a 5-year impact factor of 1.69, compared to the Journal of General Internal Medicine, which has a 5-year impact factor of 3.60.

The *American Journal of Rhinology & Allergy* offers an expedited review service for time-sensitive material; the fee for this service is $750 and is not refunded if the manuscript is rejected. The *World Journal of Gastroenterology* has four tiers of processing charges ranging from $1365 to $3000; the higher the fee paid, the quicker the turnaround time [29]. According to online respondents to the article previously cited, a "fast track for a fee" is also an option with *Current Eye Research*, *Urology*, and the *Journal of Internet Medical Research* [29].

To their credit, the NEJM, JAMA, and *Annals of Internal Medicine* all offer expedited review and publication of manuscripts describing information that might jeopardize the health of patients if the usual (i.e., slower) review and publication process is followed. Expedited review is based on the approval of the editor; there is no fee for this service.

Why Do My Manuscripts Keep Getting Rejected?

We all hate when our research report, review article, or book proposal is rejected based on peer review. It is like a friend telling us our baby is ugly. I interview applicants to Eastern Virginia Medical School, and having been part of the medical school admissions process for almost four decades, I have seen some applicants rejected several times over 2 or 3 years, only to be finally admitted and turn out to be class stars and later excellent physicians. Perhaps, in fact, there is something learned in the process of rejection and reapplication, or, in the case of written works, revision and resubmission.

In writing here about rejection, I want to present some ideas that are keys to success and some recommendations that are not included in every discussion of article rejection by peer review. Here are some key issues that can trigger rejection:

Is It True?

In the second century BCE, Claudius Galen (Fig. 5.1) told us: "We must be daring and search after Truth; even if we do not succeed in finding her, we shall at least come closer than we are at present" [30]. Reviewers, first of all, ask if what is in the paper is valid in the statistical sense. That is, are the conclusions consistent with the

Fig. 5.1 Galen of
Pergamon, the leading
clinical scientist of
classical antiquity [48]

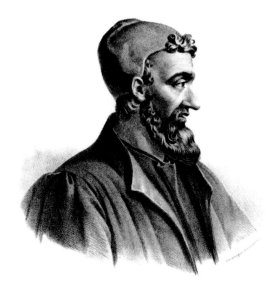

data presented and today's state of knowledge as reflected in current literature? This search for truth can present challenges. In an academic world where there is intense pressure to publish, the research team may be tempted to examine data from various perspectives, hoping to find something with a statistically significant p value. Academicians call this "data mining." But will publication of this finding bring us closer to truth?

Was the Reported Study Well Designed?

No amount of writing expertise can fix a flawed research study. In reviewing articles about what peer reviewers look for and what they reject, a recurring problem is the *Methods* section [31–33]. This is the part of the paper telling who you studied and what you did to them. There may be sample bias, inadequate numbers of subjects studied, or just plain poor study design [34]. If so, publication of the report was doomed early in the process by poor research planning.

Is the Paper Well Written?

In a world where the best journals accept a fraction of submitted papers, authors can never assume that their study is so earth-shaking that how it is written does not matter. In my role as an occasional peer reviewer, I find wordiness to be a prime offender.

The author writes four words when one will do, and uses the thesaurus for much more than avoiding duplicate wording. Pierson cites the following paragraph (author anonymous) as a humorous example of wordiness [32]: It also contains a few amusing neologisms.

> In promulgating your esoteric cogitations or articulating your superficial sentimentalities and amicable philosophical and psychological observations beware of platitudinous ponderosities. Let your communications possess a clarified conciseness, a coefficient consistency and a concatenated cogency. Eschew conglomerations of flatulated garrulity, jejune babblement and asinine affectations. Let your extemporaneous descantings and unpremeditated expatiations have intelligibility and veracious vivacity without rodomontade or thrasonical bombast. Sedulously avoid polysyllabic profundity, setatious vacuity, ventriloqual verbosity, and vain vapidity either obscurant or apparent. Shun double entendre, prurient jocosity, and pestiferous profanity.

Is the Article Written in Proper English?

Here is a problem not often addressed. The author who has learned English as a second or even third language is likely to be at a disadvantage in peer review. Persons whose native language is not English may omit articles such as "the" and fail to use plurals in the accepted English style. Idioms will not come easily. Sentences may seem tortured to the reviewer, who may make assumptions about the study based on the grammar and syntax. There are a number of services available to help English-challenged authors buff their papers prior to journal submission, and the use of them is becoming more common. To find them, Google the phrase: "non-English speaking author in scientific journals."

Does the Paper Say Anything of Current Interest?

Is anyone even going to open a journal, thumb to this paper, and read it? Papers titled "A description of our semester-long writing class at our medical school" or "A report of how our residents feel about adding behavioral science topics to the curriculum" may have been publishable a generation ago but not now—except perhaps in a predatory journal after paying a sizeable fee. Work that is too parochial, too insignificant, and too duplicative of already published science will be rejected by reputable journals.

Is There a Willingness to Revise the Manuscript to Address Reviewer Concerns?

Pierson [32] lists revision failure as one to the top reasons articles are not published. This seems to represent project burnout. After the many months of research and writing, a review arriving after a few weeks or months of waiting and then suggesting a number of revisions can be mind numbing. By that time, the researchers have gone on to other grants and studies. The team may even have drifted apart. The paper goes in a drawer while distracted investigators ponder possible revisions — and never gets out of the drawer.

What's Special About Reports of Original Research That May Influence Publication?

Describing the results of a research study is a special type of medical writing. Here are two related truisms about the publication of reports of original research:

- In considering research reports for publication peer reviewers and editors have scant tolerance for ambiguity and creativity.
- Research reports are intended not to be *read*, but to be *published and subsequently cited.*

You may have received awards for creative writing in college, but your skills with metaphor, simile, alliteration, and onomatopoeia will be of scant value in writing the report of your research. In fact, such literary niceties would probably work against you. The framework of a research report is to tell your research question, how you set out to answer the question, what you found, and what you think about what you found. There is no place for humor or irony, and rarely for classical allusions.

The purpose of a research report is to get data out there, so your colleagues can cite it and build on it. Perhaps what you describe will eventually see translation into clinical practice. A published research report also, of course, advances your academic career. It is not intended to amuse or entertain. Thus, research reports are long on data and statistics, short on theory, and generally devoid of history, philosophy, and humor.

What Is the Single Most Important Thing I Can Do to Help My Chances with the Peer Review Process?

If you can do one thing to help you achieve success in the peer review sweepstakes, it is to become very familiar with the target journal and its Instructions to Authors. Let's assume that you are a urologist and your favorite journal is the *Journal of Urology*, which happens to be the official journal of the American Urological Association. You have published several articles in this journal. But you have pioneered an image-guided method of eradicating bladder tumors and you want to publish your findings in the *Journal of Endourology*, although you have read this publication only from time to time.

In this instance, you should carefully review the latest issues of this target journal. You want to make your submission look like the reports they usually publish.

You want the reviewers to think, even subconsciously, "This seems a lot like the reports we usually publish. Let's take a good, close look at this paper."

To achieve this goal your paper should be similar to those usually published in regard to length, organization, how the abstract is constructed, the number and presentation of tables and figures, and the writing style. You are unlikely to achieve this goal by just reading the Instructions to Authors. You have to study the journal and its content.

What Is Different About Peer Review of a Review Article?

Reputable journals publish review articles as well as research reports. Most are somehow presentations of the state of the art, describing recent advances, current controversy, and hints of what the future may bring. Examples of review articles in top journals are "Treatment Of Hepatitis C: A Systematic Review" in the August 13, 2014, issue of JAMA [35] and "Kidney Transplantation In Children" in the August 7, 2014, issue of NEJM [36]. By identifying gaps in our knowledge, review articles can sometimes suggest research opportunities. Also, authors publishing review articles stake a claim to primacy in the field.

When considering a review article, peer reviewers look for some special attributes. In addition to looking at factual accuracy, appeal to the journal's audience, and proper writing, reviewers will assess whether or not the article takes "the discussion of the topic in a novel direction" [37]. As an example, the reviewer instructions for *PLOS Genetics* ask if the manuscript specifically highlights the following [37]:

- The importance of new advances in the field?
- Any remaining open questions?
- Controversies or paradoxes (where they exist)?

Reviewers will also assess the thoroughness and timeliness of the review. Do the cited references cover the full spectrum of today's work in the field? Are there any new developments not represented in the reference list? Is the lead author's work overrepresented? Are there any conspicuous omissions on the list of citations?

Publishing a review article is a good way to make a scholarly contribution without getting a grant, dealing with your institution's human subject committee, recruiting subjects, and all the rest. But don't expect peer review of your submission to be any less rigorous than that of a research report.

Can Anything Be Good About Rejection?

When your paradigm-changing paper is rejected by *The New Luminary Journal of Medicine*, remember that editors, based on reviewer comments, don't reject medical authors; they reject articles submitted to them. That is, the fact that your paper does not meet their editorial needs at this time should not diminish your self-confidence. Nor does it mean that your paper is bad. It is just not "right" for that journal.

Now doesn't that make you feel better?

What Is Probably the Top Reason a Manuscript Is Never Published?

In the study of top ten reasons why manuscripts are not published, Pierson lists the top reason as this: The paper is never written. He cites a study by Weber et al. of blinded reviews of abstracts submitted to an emergency medicine meeting in 1991, and then followed up to how many had resulted in a publication over the next 5 years. A questionnaire sent to abstract authors showed that of the authors of abstracts, only 20 % had gone on to prepare and submit a manuscript to a peer-reviewed journal [32, 38].

How Can I Find a Publisher for a Book I Want to Write?

Your first decision is whether you are planning to write a professional/medical reference book or textbook versus a trade book. What you are reading is a medical book, even though there are no diseases and drugs described; it was written for a professional audience. The other genre is the trade book, written for the general public, whether or not the subject is "medical." Doctor Jerome Groopman's book *How Doctors Think* [39] is as much a trade book as the Harry Potter series. The publishers of the two genres—professional vs. trade books—are quite different and, even when under the umbrella of the same large company, they are separate divisions who seldom communicate. Curiously, finding a publisher for a trade book is much more difficult than achieving publication of a professional book.

Whichever type of book you plan, the right pathway is this: Start with a proposal that includes a letter describing the book you plan to write, why you are qualified to write the book, how long the manuscript will be, an estimate of the number of tables and figures (if any), any competing competitors and why your book will be different and better, and, very important, who will buy your book. Append the following items to your letter:

- A table of contents, perhaps with a short annotation of what each chapter will cover.
- A sample chapter, to show that you can string words together without getting tangled.
- Your curriculum vitae.

Then send your proposal packet off electronically. If proposing a professional book, send your packet to a medical publisher, such as Springer, who publishes my writing books. If proposing a trade book and hoping for robust sales, you may want to skip the anguish and frustration of contacting a publisher directly; most major publishers will only consider books submitted by an agent. And so you will need to find an agent, also not an easy endeavor.

If planning a professional book, I suggest that you stop here and do not finish the book, especially if your book will contain time-sensitive, rapidly evolving information. If and when your proposal is accepted, the book editor and publisher will have a lot to say about what they think should be covered and how it should be approached. By waiting until you have signed a contract before moving ahead with the unwritten chapters, you may save yourself a lot of unnecessary rewriting to deal with their recommendations. Having said this, I have found some authors of trade books who recommend writing the entire book before seeking publication.

Readers tempted to go the book writing route and who want to know more are referred to Chap. 8: "Writing Book Chapters and Books" in my book *Medical Writing: a Guide for Clinicians, Educators, and Researchers*, 2nd edition [40].

Should I Self-Publish My Book?

The bestseller *Fifty Shades of Gray* by British author E.L. James was initially self-published, and subsequently picked up by a major publisher [41, 42]. James was not the first author to underwrite the publication of his or her work. There is a rich history of self-publishing in the English-speaking world. Benjamin Franklin's *Poor Richard's Almanac* was self-published (after all, Franklin's trade was printing, which surely was an advantage), as was Thomas Paine's *Common Sense*. Other well-known authors who self-published some of their writings were Willa Cather, Herman Melville, and Mark Twain [43].

I don't know of any noteworthy medical reference or textbooks that have been self-published. Many physicians have the urge to write, and there have been a number of self-published books describing the experiences and accumulated wisdom of physician authors. Some are philosophical; others tell of case histories or the authors' contributions to medicine. One of these is the recently published *40 Years in Family Medicine*, an anthology of previously published articles by Joseph E. Scherger, MD [44]. The publisher is listed as CreateSpace Independent Publishing Platform, which is owned by Amazon Bookstore. Marketing is always an issue with self-publication; Scherger's self-published book is readily available to a wide audience on Amazon.com.

There are more than new 20,000 self-published books released each week [45]. As we see the creation of more and more legitimate publish-your-own-book companies and with the advent of online transmission of manuscripts and pages, self-publishing is losing the stigma it once endured. That distain is now more appropriately directed toward predatory journals. Still, I continue to think that the best use of self-publishing is for autobiographies, personal reflections, and family histories, books for which a large commercial audience is not anticipated.

My Article Manuscript or Book Proposal Has Been Rejected for the Fifth Time: What Should I Do Now?

No publisher seems to want your work. Should you give up or keep trying? The answer to this question may have more to do with your state of mind than your writing.

Consider some of medicine's giants who faced initial rejection. In the late eighteenth century, the Royal Society of London initially rejected Edward Jenner's original paper on his use of cowpox vaccination to prevent smallpox. Following revisions, the paper was eventually published.

Following his discovery in 1848 that hand washing could reduce the incidence of childbed fever, Ignaz Semmelweis wrote to his colleague describing what he had learned. His findings were finally published in a 1858 monograph titled *The Etiology of Childbed Fever*. Semmelweis found that his work was not only scorned by peers; his colleagues and his wife, believing him to be insane, had him committed to an asylum, where he died 2 weeks later.

There have been a number of scientific papers that were initially rejected and yet went on to help earn their authors the Nobel Prize (see Fig. 5.2). In 1937 the paper by Hans Krebs describing the citric acid cycle that we now know as the Krebs cycle was rejected by *Nature*. The paper by Krebs was later published in *Enzymologia*. In 1986 Stanley Cohen's work on growth factor earned him a Nobel Prize; but an early article on the topic was initially rejected. The report by Kary Mullis describing the polymerase chain reaction as a method for analyzing DNA was initially rejected by both *Nature* and *Science*; based on the work described in his writing Mullis was a 1993 Nobel Laureate [46].

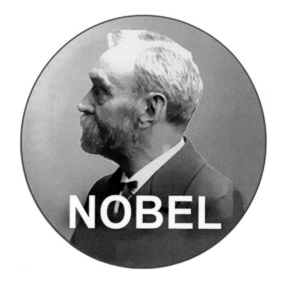

Fig. 5.2 Alfred Nobel, Swedish chemist and inventor of dynamite, whose will left funds that established the Nobel Prize [49]

In the field of popular literature, American author Jack London received 600 rejections before he sold his first story. Beatrix Potter received numerous rejections, became discouraged with commercial publishing houses, and initially self-published *The Tale of Peter Rabbit*. Louis L'Amour had 200 rejections before seeing his first book in print. Doubleday rejected Dan Brown's *The Da Vinci Code*, describing it as "badly written." Twelve publishers rejected J.K. Rowling's book about a wizard boy named Harry Potter, until an editor's 8-year-old daughter picked up the book and wouldn't let it go [47].

The message to medical writers is this. Don't become discouraged with the first, second, or third rejection. Your article may not earn you a Noble Prize, your book may never make the best-seller list, but—perhaps with some revision—it may be publishable.

References

1. Ware M et al. An overview of scientific and scholarly journal publishing. STM Rep. http://www.stm-assoc.org/2012_12_11_STM_Report_2012.pdf.
2. Jinha A. Article 50 million: an estimate of the number of scholarly articles in existence. Learn Publ. 2010;23:258.
3. Wasserman L. Letter. Wall St J. 19 July 2014, p A10.
4. Smith R. The trouble with medical journals. J R Soc Med. 2006;99:115.
5. Peters DP, Ceci SJ. Peer-review practices of psychological journals: the fate of published articles, submitted again. Behav Brain Sci. 1982;5:187.
6. US Department of Health and Human Services. National Institutes of Health Public Access. Updated 2013. http://publicaccess.nih.gov.
7. Berner ES. Publications in academic medical centers: technology-facilitated culture clash. Acad Med. 2010;89:1.
8. Irwin D et al. Opinion: learning from peer review. Scientist. http://www.the-scientist.com/?articles.view/articleNo/35608/title/Opinion–Learning-from-Peer-Review/.
9. Rockwell S. Ethics of peer review: a guide for manuscript reviewers. http://radonc.yale.edu/Images/Ethical_Issues_in_Peer_Review_tcm307-34211.pdf.
10. Nyberg AK. Understanding the book proposal review process. Academic Coaching and Writing. http://www.academiccoachingandwriting.org/academic-coaching/cc-blog/vi-understanding-the-book-proposal-review-process/.
11. Bauchner H, et al. To JAMA authors, peer reviewers, and readers – thank you. JAMA. 2015;313:675.
12. Ingersoll KS, et al. Publishing HIV/AIDS behavioural science reports: an author's guide. AIDS Care. 2006;18:674.
13. Whoriskey P. As drug industry's influence over research grows, so does the potential for bias. Wash Post. http://www.washingtonpost.com/business/economy/as-drug-industrys-influence-over-research-grows-so-does-the-potential-for-bias/2012/11/24/bb64d596-1264-11e2-be82-c3411b7680a9_story.html.
14. Washington H. Flacking for big pharma. American Scholar. http://theamericanscholar.org/flacking-for-big-pharma/#.Uxx6e-ddWQ0.
15. Kesselheim AS, et al. A randomized study of how physicians interpret research funding disclosures. N Engl J Med. 2012;367:1119.
16. Ross JS, et al. Time to publication among completed clinical trials. JAMA Intern Med. 2013;173:825.
17. Gordon D, et al. Publication of trials funded by the National Heart, Lung, and Blood Institute. N Engl J Med. 2013;369:1926.

18. Why publish in JAMA? JAMA Network. http://jama.jamanetwork.com/public/WhyPublish. aspx.
19. About Gut. http://gut.bmj.com/site/about/.
20. Frank M. Open but not free – publishing in the 21st century. N Engl J Med. 2013;368:787.
21. PLOS ONE celebrates milestone. http://www.plos.org/plos-celebrates-milestone/.
22. 2013 Journal citation reports science edition. Philadelphia: Thompson Reuters; 2014.
23. Huag C. The downside of open access publishing. N Engl J Med. 2013;368:791.
24. Beall J. Predatory publishers are corrupting open access. Nature. 2012;489:179.
25. Bohannon J. Who's afraid of peer review? Science. 2013;342:60. http://www.sciencemag.org/content/342/6154/60.full.
26. Beale J. List of predatory publishers. Scholarly Open Access. http://scholarlyoa.com/2014/01/02/list-of-predatory-publishers-2014/.
27. Rennie D. Quoted in: Smith JS. The trouble with medical journals. Medico-Legal J. 2008;76:79.
28. Instructions for authors. Postgrad Med. https://postgradmed.org/authors.
29. Want a faster review? Pay for it. Scholarly Open Access. http://scholarlyoa.com/2013/11/07/want-a-faster-review-pay-for-it/.
30. McDonald P. Oxford dictionary of medical quotations. New York: Oxford University Press; 2004, p. 38.
31. Byrne DW. Common reasons for rejecting manuscripts at medical journals: a survey of editors and peer reviewers. Sci Ed. 2000;23:39. http://www.udel.edu/chs/atep/downloads/Common Reasons for Rejecting Manuscripts.pdf.
32. Pierson DJ. The top 10 reasons why manuscripts are not accepted for publication. Resp Care. 2004;49:1246.
33. Thrower P. Eight reasons I rejected your article. Elsevierconnect. http://www.elsevier.com/connect/8-reasons-i-rejected-your-article.
34. Taylor RB. How to write a report of a clinical study. In: Taylor RB, editor. Medical writing: a guide for clinicians, educators, and researchers. 2nd ed. New York: Springer; 2011, p. 276.
35. Kohli A, et al. Treatment of hepatitis C: a systematic review. JAMA. 2014;312:631.
36. Dharnidharka VR, et al. Kidney transplantation in children. N Engl J Med. 2014;371:549.
37. Peer review of viewpoints and review articles. ITEM 6. PLOS Genet Guidel Reviewers. http://www.plosgenetics.org/static/reviewerGuidelines#frontmatter.
38. Weber EJ, et al. Unpublished research from a medical specialty meeting: why investigators fail to publish. JAMA. 1998;280:257.
39. Groopman J. How doctors think. New York: Scribe; 2010.
40. Taylor RB. Writing book chapters and books. In: Medical writing: a guide for clinicians, educators, and researchers. 2nd ed. New York: Springer; 2011, p 189.
41. James EL. 50 Shades of gray. New York: Vintage; 2012.
42. Altucher J. 21 things you need to know about self-publishing 2.0. http://www.copyblogger.com/professional-self-publishing/.
43. Fay S. After "Fifty shades of gray," what's next for self-publishing? Atlantic. http://www.theatlantic.com/entertainment/archive/2012/04/after-fifty-shades-of-grey-whats-next-for-self-publishing/255338/. Accessed 2 Apr 2012.
44. Scherger JE. 40 Years in family medicine. Printed by CreateSpace Independent Publishing Platform. 2014.
45. Tomaselli KP. Writing your way to a bigger physician brand. Am Med News. http://www.amednews.com/article/20130902/business/130909995/4/.
46. Campanario JM et al. Rejecting Nobel class article and resisting Nobel class discoveries. http://www.uah.es/otrosweb/jmc/.
47. Best-sellers initially rejected. Lit Rejections. http://www.literaryrejections.com/best-sellers-initially-rejected/.
48. Galen detail.jpg. Galen of Pergamon. This work is in the public domain. http://commons.wikimedia.org/wiki/File:Galen_detail.jpg.
49. Nobel.png, Alfred Nobel. This work is in the public domain. http://commons.wikimedia.org/wiki/File:NobelP.png.

Chapter 6
Ethical Issues in Medical Writing

There are a number of ethical issues in the practice of medicine. These include confidentiality (the sanctity of what the patient tells the physician), beneficence (the imperative to do good for the patient), non-maleficence (doing nothing to harm the patient, as admonished by Hippocrates), justice (being fair to all involved), informed consent (being sure the patient knows what is about to happen), and simple honesty (even if it means admitting an error).

Medical writing has its own ethical issues, many of which revolve around the preparation of research reports for publication. Those we will cover in this chapter include the following: Who is an author and who, in fact, is a contributor? Who owns the rights to published material? What constitutes plagiarism and when do I need to worry about it? What are the ethics of submitting works for publication? What about the so-called ghostwriting? What constitutes conflict of interest, either intellectual or financial? And, as if there would be any questions about the ethics involved, what writing assignments skirt the law or are outright fraudulent publications?

What Are Important Ethical Issues in Authorship?

The development of "new knowledge" represents the pinnacle of achievement in academic medicine, and the formal recognition is authorship of an important article published in a prestigious scholarly journal, linking the author's name to a noteworthy discovery, insight, or solution. A single groundbreaking paper can supercharge an academic career. For these reasons, identifying who is and who is not an author, and especially the lead author, becomes important.

In the case of a published research report, the most frequent locus of ethical issues is in regard to who qualifies to have their name in print. At the core of the issue, an

© Springer International Publishing Switzerland 2015
R.B. Taylor, *What Every Medical Writer Needs to Know*,
DOI 10.1007/978-3-319-20264-8_6

"author" is someone who made significant contributions to a study, participated in writing the report, and who understands and stands behind the submitted manuscript [1]. Although this seems quite straightforward, ethical issues arise in three main areas: honorary authorship, anonymous authorship, and first authorship.

Honorary Authorship

You may see the terms "honorary," "courtesy," or even "gift" authorship. Using the term "undeserved coauthorship," Wislar et al. surveyed the authors of articles in six respected high-impact general medical journals. These included *Nature Medicine* and the *Journal of the American Medical Association* (JAMA). They found evidence of honorary or ghost authorship in 21 % of the articles in the study sample [2].

Slone surveyed the first authors of 275 research reports published in the *American Journal of Radiology* [3]. Here is what was found:

- Criteria defining authorship were contributions to research design, data collection, data analysis, and manuscript preparation. Of those who were third author and beyond, only one-third could meet three of the four criteria.
- The more authors on a paper, the more undeserved coauthors. In papers with more than six authors the incidence of undeserved authors was 30 %.
- The incidence of undeserved coauthorship was 45 % when the first author was non-tenured versus 28 % when the first author was tenured.
- Only 80 % of manuscripts in the study had been read by all the authors.
- Only 78 % of all authors were considered by the lead author respondents to understand the manuscript sufficiently to defend it before an audience of peers.

The most common reason undeserving coauthors are listed is the quest for academic promotion, although, according to Slone, "obligation" or "fear" may sometimes play a role [3]. If my department chair's name is not added to the author list, will he or she back me when it comes time for promotion? We might well call this authorship by guilt or intimidation.

A 2014 study of 109 articles from 102 journals revealed honor authors in 8.3 % and authors with insufficient contribution in 46.8 %. They also found that 6.4 % of papers had evidence of ghost authorship, discussed below [4].

At least for those in an academic setting, honorary authorship is not simply a harmless "gift." The practice compromises the standards for academic appointments, and diminishes the respect for those who have honestly earned senior faculty status.

In Chap. 7, in the setting of some tongue-in-cheek literary awards, I will present the award for most egregious instance of author inflation: The Most Authors on a Single Paper Award.

Anonymous Authorship

Anonymous authorship, aka ghost authorship, seems the obverse of honorary authorship. In anonymous writing, the author receives no acknowledgement at all for the work done. By ghost authorship, I mean the practice of writing—composing, revising, and completing—a manuscript without putting one's name on it, allowing someone else to have that "honor." Pharmaceutical companies employ many of these anonymous medical writers.

In my research I came across an article written by Linda Logdberg, whom I would describe as a recovering ghostwriter [5]. She describes writing journal articles, continuing medical education (CME) programs, monographs, and more. She tells of, for the most part, never seeing the finished paper, "nor did [she] care to" [5].

But Logdberg's work was published, and someone else's name was on it as author. Who was listed as author? Fugh-Berman describes how "the pharmaceutical company Wyeth used ghost-written articles to mitigate the perceived risks of breast cancer" associated with menopausal hormone replacement therapy. She describes some 1500 such articles, and tells how the attributed "author" might offer suggestions to the final manuscript, and how such changes might or might not be accepted, depending on their perceived effect on the advertising message [6].

The editors of *PLOS Medicine* tell of a instance in which a major pharmaceutical manufacturer had a manuscript "written and approved" but had, at the time the email described was written, "received no word on authors for the … manuscript." Thus, it seems that a report had been ghostwritten and "approved," and now the pharmaceutical company was searching for professionals with some academic credentials willing to serve as guest authors [7].

Logdberg sums it up well: "Yet advertising masquerading as unbiased health information clearly threatens the fundamental assumptions of scientific research" [5]. Despite criticism, the practice of anonymous authorship funded by pharmaceutical dollars continues because the financial stakes are enormous. The ethics of medical ghostwriting are debated, at least as far as the actions of the writer are concerned. But, in the view of the European Medical Writers Association, for a scientist or physician to lend his or her name to a ghostwritten article, claiming authorship in print and taking responsibility for research without being a part of it, is clearly a breech of professional ethics [8].

Guest authorship represents such an insult to academic credibility that some journals have advocated formal retraction of any report in which there was proven guest authorship, a ban on future publication of submissions by any known guest author, and informing the guest author's institution of his or her unethical actions [5].

First Authorship

In an ideal world there would be no issues regarding the order of authors listed on a published research report. But such controversies arise all too often, and become an ethical issue when the final listing of authors occurs because of power, prestige, intimidation, or gratitude. In fact, listing a primary author for any reason other than evidence of leadership on the project, typically serving as principal investigator (PI), is a breech of ethics.

How much does it matter? Just look at my personal shorthand method of citing publications, listing only the first author followed by "et al" if there are more. The reference lists of my latest issue of the *New England Journal of Medicine* identify the first three authors, followed by "et al" if more than three. The International Council of Medical Journal Editors (ICMJE) prescribes listing up to six authors and adding "et al" if there are more than six [9].

Thus, being lead author (when deserved) is best, and if not, you should at least try to be in the first three listed. Being author number seven or eight may banish your involvement to "et al" anonymity.

Being lead author of a paper becomes critically important when the time comes for promotion and tenure (P&T) consideration. The P&T Committee logically assumes that the first author is actually the PI who developed the research idea, assembled and managed the team, and took the lead in writing the report. That is how it is supposed to happen. Furthermore, it would seem logical that subsequent authors would be listed according to their contribution to the project. But in a survey of 919 corresponding authors of published research reports, more than two-thirds disputed the contributions claimed by their coauthors [10].

Conflict may arise when the real work has been done by someone outranked by others on the team, when the team believes that listing a certain name as first author will increase chances of publication, or that—believe it or not—the research team assigns first authorship to a lessor contributor in a magnanimous gesture to promote this person's academic advancement.

One compromise might be to designate *co-first-authorship* in instances when two authors have contributed equally to the project. The first two authors may have an asterisk next to their names to indicate that they are both coauthors. I recently found an example: A paper on the comparative effectiveness of high-dose versus standard-dose influenza vaccines in older Americans has two lead authors, designated as: "These authors contributed equally" [11]. I play poker and this feels to me like splitting a pot when two hands are equal.

Although it may sound a little too simple, I believe that the best way to avoid first-authorship and order-of-author issues is to have a frank discussion early in the project, not waiting until the third draft of the report.

What About Professional Medical Writers Assisting Investigator-Authors in Developing an Article for a Peer-Reviewed Publication?

I hope that many readers of this book will be professional medical writers, the people who help make research reports, review articles, advertising copy, and reports to the Food and Drug Administration (FDA) the best they can be. Some medical schools employ professional writers/editors to help assure that papers submitted from their institutions for publication are of the highest quality. Many professional medical writers are employed in the pharmaceutical or medical device industry to improve the prose of medical professionals. These persons differ from ghostwriters in that they *assist* authors rather than creating reports for someone else to claim authorship.

The work of the professional medical writer is often recognized in some way in the paper. In fact the European Medical Writers Association (EMWA) advocates that this routinely be done: "The involvement of medical writers and their source of funding should be acknowledged. Identifying the writer, either as an author or contributor or in the acknowledgement section, helps readers, reviewers, and journal editors to understand how the manuscript was developed and recognize the writer's involvement" [8].

Who Owns the Rights to Published Material That I Have Written?

The domain of ethical issues in writing includes who owns the words you have written and the figures you have created, and who can use them.

According to the US Copyright Law of 1978, copyright protection begins when a work—article, book, and even a song—is created and fixed in a "copy or phonorecord for the first time" [12]. Registration of copyright protection to your work is added insurance, but probably unnecessary. Why? Because the publisher of your scientific article or book will generally copyright the book in its own name. For most scholarly works, copyright protection lasts for 70 years from the time of creation.

Thus the chapter you are reading was protected by copyright the day the book was printed. The publisher, Springer, holds the copyright. If I had been somehow concerned and did not want to wait for the book to be published, I could have printed a copy of the chapter, tagged it with "Copyright, Robert B. Taylor, 2016," and distributed it to participants in a writing seminar. Subsequently I would have assigned the rights to the publisher.

Do I Need to Apply for Copyright for My Own Work?

In almost all instances, seeking copyright registration of your work is unnecessary. Your publisher will handle this for you. You are in little danger of anyone stealing your work, especially in view of today's sophisticated programs to detect plagiarism.

Your greater danger is having someone appropriate your ideas. In academic medicine, your greatest asset can be a *good idea*, such as a "eureka" researchable hypothesis, an unanticipated clinical finding that may change how we approach disease, or a concept for a publishable article or book. If you are blessed with such a good idea, nurture it carefully and share it with caution.

When Do I Need to Ask for Permission
for the Use of Borrowed Material?

Part of the answer is easy. You need permission to reproduce any previously published table or figure. You also need permission to "adapt" any table or figure. Changing something just a little doesn't make it "yours." If you combine bits of data from four studies to create your own table or figure, I think that the creation is yours and no permission is needed; but you should identify your data sources in the table or figure legend. Your editor may disagree with my opinion about tables or figures created from multiple published studies and require that you seek permissions from all sources.

The next gray issue is the use of text (phrases, sentences, and paragraphs) from published sources. All borrowed work, even a few words, should be attributed to the source. This protects you from allegations of theft. You borrowed the words and told where you got them.

When borrowing a few sentences or more, when do you need to seek permission for use? This is a bit of a legal Neverland, and the answer is not nearly as clear as with tables and figures. The legal doctrine involves "fair use" and you will see allusions to needing permission to borrow "lengthy quotations." What constitutes "fair use" and how long is a "lengthy quotation?" Section 107 of the Copyright Act lists four factors considered in fair-use issues [13, 14]:

- The nature of the use, including whether commercial or nonprofit.
- The nature of the copyrighted work.
- How much of the work is used in relation to the whole.
- Any possible effect on the future value of the copyrighted work.

Very rarely does a legal issue arise when credit is given for reasonable use of borrowed words. Allegations of plagiarism are one thing; legal complaints are quite another, and are unlikely when the author has used a quotation with careful attribution to the source. We do not have chiseled-in-stone definitions of *fair use* and *lengthy quotation*; "fair" and "lengthy" may depend on how much of the work is quoted. If a dispute arises, all legal issues are ultimately settled by negotiated agreement or trial. Court decisions have described fair use as including "short passages of a scholarly or technical work, for illustration or clarification of the author's observations" and "reproduction by a teacher or student of a small part of a work to illustrate a lesson" [14]. I will go out on a limb and state that you should seek permission if you are quoting more than 150 words, even with attribution.

In this book, I have often used direct quotations, especially when stating something that might be controversial and I wanted to be sure I presented things correctly. I don't think any of my borrowed, and carefully attributed, quotations (such as the Dizzy Awards in Chap. 4) will adversely affect the future value of the original copyrighted work. In fact, they may prompt the reader to search out and read the original article or buy the book cited. The length and attribution of all quotations in this book are such that I did not seek any permissions for use.

While on the topic of borrowed material, some items not protected by copyright include slogans, short phrases, and data that are considered common and authorless property such as standard calendars, height and weight charts, and tape measures and rulers.

What About Borrowing Illustrations and Text to Use in My Lectures?

Academicians have long appropriated material from books and websites to use in their PowerPoint (PPT) lectures. Although perhaps a copyright infringement, the "harm" to the copyright holder has been negligible and complaints were rare. But things are changing.

Today PPT lectures and transcripts are posted on the Web and what was once a talk given to a few dozen students has become an illustrated presentation available to thousands at distant sites. Another factor in this change is the "flipped classroom," in which students view an online lecture before class and use classroom time for discussion. This means that what was once a trivial case of borrowing words and illustrations for limited classroom use has become a minefield of possible copyright violations. Each of the many colorful illustrations you find online probably belongs to someone, and if you appropriate the wrong one, you may hear from a lawyer. Beware even the copyrighted cartoon. Recently, some academic institutions have been sued after teachers included copyrighted items in their Web-based lectures without seeking proper permission [15].

Here is an example of what medical educators may face. In 2008, three publishers sued Georgia State University, claiming that faculty members went beyond fair use in material posted online for students, alleging 99 copyright infringements. In May, 2012, a long 4 years later, a federal judge in Atlanta ruled in favor of Georgia State University in all but five of the allegations. But the five allegations in which the publishers prevailed should serve as a warning to all who post lectures online [16].

Are There Illustrations I Can Use for My Lectures and Other Works That Are Free of Copyright Protection, and Where Can I Find Them?

Yes, there are online sites presenting figures that you can use freely, with proper attribution. Most of these are in the public domain, many because they are classic works that have long outlived any copyright protection. An example in this book is the illustration of Hippocrates (Fig. 1.2). Or sometimes the figure has been published for us under the Creative Commons Attribution 3.0 Unported license; an example is the image of medical author Abraham Verghese (Fig. 2.2).

My favorite site for finding illustrations that may be helpful in your writing is Wikimedia Commons. Many images here are in the public domain for reasons such as a copyright that has expired, creation by a US Government employee as part of his or her employment, or specific release by the copyright owner into the public domain.

Do I Need Permission to Use Material from US Government Publications and Websites?

No. All material in government publications may be used without seeking permission. Nevertheless, careful authors always give full credit to the source, even if it is the US Government.

Can I Rely on the Accuracy of Reference Citations and Quotations in Published Medical Articles?

In a word, no. This is just one reason why you must cite only original sources you have viewed. Whether intentionally or not, authors often present misleading interpretations of material from references cited in articles and books. The problem often arises when the author relies on a secondary source for what was previously reported, even if the secondary source lists a plausible reference site.

Some bibliographic errors have been humorous. In 1887 Czech author Jaroslav Hlava wrote an article titled "O Uplavici;" in the author's language, the title means "on dysentery." When the article was subsequently abstracted in a German medical journal, the author's name was listed as O. Uplavici [17]. Misspelled author names and incorrect journal citations sometimes make sources impossible to check.

But the problem extends beyond clumsy presentation of reference citations. Misquotation is not uncommon in scientific articles. In a study by de Lacey et al., a review of articles published in six medical journals showed "The original author was misquoted in 15 % of all references, and most of the errors would have misled readers. Errors in citation of references occurred in 24 %, of which 8 % were major errors—that is, they prevented immediate identification of the source of the reference" [18].

While we, as charitable readers, might consider the inaccurate presentation of reference citations as simple carelessness, the misquotation of original authors in scientific publications seems more likely to represent an effort to mislead the writer's audience, which would clearly be an ethical transgression.

Can We At Least Trust the Data Found in Reports of Randomized Clinical Trials?

The randomized clinical trial (RCT), the foundation of new scholarly knowledge and the pinnacle of scientific achievement for the author, might sometimes merit a second look. Ebrahim et al. examined instances in which raw data from RCTs reported in the literature were subjected to reanalysis [19].

From a comprehensive MEDLINE database, they found 37 eligible reanalyses of raw data in 36 published articles, with only a small number of second looks conducted by scientists not involved in the original study.

The good news is that in 65 % of studies, the reassessment confirmed the findings and conclusions originally reported. The worrisome news is that 35 % of reanalyses "led to changes in findings that implied conclusions different from those of the original article about the types and number of patients that should be treated" [19].

Is Plagiarism a Problem in Medical Writing Today?

A notice of retraction posted in the December 2010 issue of the journal *Anesthesia and Analgesia* described how the editorial staff had discovered that a paper they had recently published—"The Effect of Celiac Plexus Block in Critically Ill Patients Intolerant of Enteral Nutrition: A Randomized, Placebo-Controlled Study"—had been, in part, plagiarized from other manuscripts. The published notice goes further and, to be sure I get it right (and don't plagiarize), I am going to quote directly: "The retraction would have been fairly mundane, if still somewhat disappointing, if it had not been for a separate request for retraction in the same issue. In that request for retraction, an Indian physician requested that a manuscript he had contributed be retracted due to the discovery of plagiarized material inside it. That, too, would be uninteresting if it weren't for the fact that the Indian paper was one of the five papers cited in the retraction for the first. Meaning that the first paper was retracted, in part, for plagiarizing from a paper that was retracted for plagiarism" [20]. You just can't make this up.

According to the same report cited above, the journal *Cancer Biology and Therapy* "rejected 211 article submissions for plagiarism in 2012" [20]. I don't know how many manuscripts are submitted to this well-regarded journal (Impact Factor 3.63) each year, but 211 papers with plagiarized text seems to be a lot. I wonder how many of these found their way into print in other journals after initial rejection by *Cancer Biology and Therapy*.

According to Roig, there are specific types of intellectual theft: *Plagiarism of text* describes simply copying someone else's written work and submitting it as your own [21]. *Plagiarism of ideas* describes appropriating concepts from someone else's conference presentation or even a paper one has been asked to review. Appropriation of the ideas of another has a long history in medical writing, and the

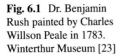

Fig. 6.1 Dr. Benjamin
Rush painted by Charles
Willson Peale in 1783.
Winterthur Museum [23]

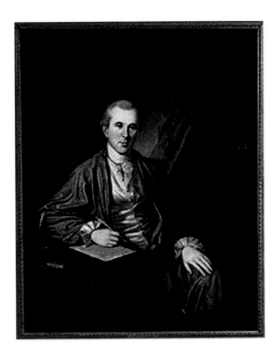

stories are generally unpleasant. Science writer Stephen Jay Gould comments,
"Debates about the priority of ideas are usually the most misdirected in the history
of science" [22]. In fairness to all, there is the truism that sometimes we see "an idea
whose time has come," and in the many conversations that occur among scientists,
unconscious adoption of a concept can occur. With that said, here are some
examples of apparently appropriated ideas.

Founding father and signer of the Declaration of Independence Benjamin Rush,
MD, was once accused of concept plagiarism (see Fig. 6.1). Rush, who held the
Chair of the Institutes of Medicine and Clinical Practice of the University of
Pennsylvania in Philadelphia, was accused in 1794 by medical student Charles
Caldwell of describing in a lecture a "hydropathic cure" of fever—immersion in
water or wetting the patient in rain—that Caldwell had previously explained to
Rush. Then in 1795 Rush went on to deliver a paper before his peers titled "Use of
Cold Water in the Treatment of Fever" [24].

In 1999, a graduate student at Columbia University sued her professor, a member
of her thesis committee, alleging that he used her ideas about teaching nutrition in a
research grant proposal and in his lectures, without giving her credit [25].

"Easy reading is damn hard writing." In Chap. 3, I cited this adage, first written
by Nathaniel Hawthorne in the mid-nineteenth century. This saying had been subsequently often repeated by twentieth-century American authors Ernest Hemingway,
Maya Angelou, and some others much less well known, and not always with attribution to Hawthorne [26]. Was this plagiarism as we understand it today, or has the
aphorism simply become part of our heritage, so that we no longer need to give credit
to the source?

The word plagiarism comes from Latin *plagiarius*, meaning kidnapper. This seems an apt name for the nefarious practice of, according to Das et al., wrongfully presenting "someone else's work or idea as one's own without adequately attributing it to the source" [27]. Just as an example, I quoted my source in the previous sentence; there is no question what words I have borrowed.

On the other hand, if I take out the quotation marks, and omit the attribution, that would be plagiarism. If I go on to change just a word or two, it would be what Das et al. call *mosaic plagiarism*: intertwining one's own ideas and opinions with the ideas, opinions, and words of an original source, without clearly acknowledging the source.

Then there is *self-plagiarism*, discussed next.

Is There Really Such a Thing as Self-Plagiarism?

If the words or data are mine, can't I use them again?

One of my favorite writers is Isaac Asimov, who authored hundreds of books and stories, many of them science fiction. An author on diverse topics, his works also included: *The Kite That Won the Revolution* (New York: Houghton Mifflin; 1963), *Asimov's Guide to Shakespeare* (New York: Random House; 1970), and *Beginnings: The Story of Origins—of Mankind, Life, the Earth, the Universe* (New York: Walker and Co.; 1989). Asimov was clearly one of America's most accomplished authors, and yet, he was known to practice what one might deem self-plagiarism. One of his most colorful quotes is this: "If my doctor told me I had only six months to live, I wouldn't brood. I'd type a little faster." This quip is found on page 51 of *How to Enjoy Writing: A Book of Aid and Comfort*, which he coauthored in 1987 with his wife Janet Asimov [28], and also, although phrased just a little differently, on page 205 of his (second) autobiography, *I. Asimov: A Memoir*, published in 1994 [29].

Some might criticize me for reusing the same tales in different books. I am fond of the stories of William Jenner and Blossom the cow, of the determined battle of Ignaz Semmelweis to convince his colleagues of the merits of hand washing, and of Sir William Osler's publication of an outrageously satirical medical article under the pseudonym Egerton Yorrick Davis. I write books on medical writing (all of the above were medical authors) and also about medical history. I have used these stories before, I present versions of them in Chap. 8 of this book, and I may use them again in the future. However, they are all familiar "white coat tales," and in each instance I tell the story a little differently, and I use it to illustrate a different point.

Self-plagiarism is widely practiced in reports of research studies, and perhaps what is described next is not a bad thing, particularly when there will be multiple reports emanating from the same major study. Writing in *Academic Medicine* in 2014, Berner describes: "Although academic medical faculty abhor plagiarizing other people's work, they may not consider the reuse of their own material to be a problem. For example, many researchers in large studies use a standard Methods section for all publications related to that study. This practice ensures clarity and consistency when discussing different aspects of the results. In addition, the introductions to various publications on the same or related studies are likely to include similar citations, if not actual repetition of text" [15]. Roig calls this "text recycling" [30].

Then there is duplicate publication, discussed next.

Does Duplicate Publication Occur in the Scientific Literature?

In 1848, the American Medical Association (AMA) held its first annual meeting. On the agenda was the report of the *AMA Committee on Medical Literature*, chaired by Oliver Wendell Holmes, Sr. (see Fig. 6.2). The Committee's report condemned the fact that many scientific reports were being published in more than one journal, stating, "The ring of editors sit in each other's laps, with perfect propriety, and great convenience it is true, but with a wonderful saving in the article of furniture" [32].

But what about today? The editors of the *Journal of General Internal Medicine* describe a paper published in their journal and then published online in a very similar form in another journal. "Both papers reported on a quasi-experimental evaluation of a quality improvement intervention. The titles, by-lines, and abstracts were similar and the methods sections almost identical. Moreover, entire paragraphs of the introduction and discussion sections were almost the same." Further investigation revealed that, although the papers described the same intervention, the settings, subjects, and study designs differed somewhat [33]. Was this truly duplicate publication? Perhaps not. But did the reuse of prior words and paragraphs call the ethics of the authors into question? Yes, I think so.

Fig. 6.2 Image of poet/ professor Oliver Wendell Holmes, Sr. with a facsimile of his autograph. From A Portrait Catalogue of the Books Published by Houghton Mifflin Company, 1906 [31]

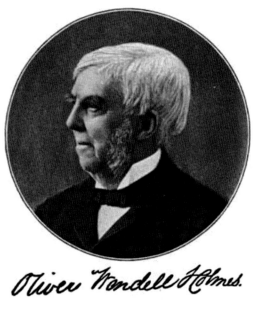

A website titled *Scholarly Open Access: Critical Analysis of Scholarly Open-Access Publishing* describes two articles on the topic of sleep patterns that were published in late 2013 and early 2014. The two articles each had six authors, of which four appeared on both reports. The site reports, "Although the titles differ, the text in the two articles is mostly the same" [34].

A study from Korea showed that of 86 published meta-analyses, 6 (6.9 %) included duplicate publications [35]. What shall we think about the conclusions of these flawed meta-analyses?

The Virginia Bioinformatics Institute maintains "Déjà vu: A Database Of Highly Similar Citations" [36]. The site presents a list of Medline citations that are "extremely similar." The authors are careful to point out: "Many, but not all, … contain instances of duplicate publication and plagiarism" [36].

Duplicate publication lowers the quality of the scientific literature and confounds the results of meta-analyses. It is a practice that should be condemned by every serious medical writer.

What About the Abstract That Was Printed Last Year in a Conference Proceedings Document? Could This Be Self-Plagiarism—A "Prior Publication"—When a Journal Article Is Later Published?

Abstracts of research presentations published in conference proceedings syllabi are important in the career advancement of academicians. They count as publications— of a sort. Some of these abstracts, occurring months before a related paper is formally published describing the research methods and conclusions, achieve wide dissemination. But is this material "self-plagiarism" when included in a later published paper? Probably not. Each journal will have a different opinion or even guidelines. A good model is described in the *Academic Medicine* Instructions for Authors: "Short abstracts (250–300 words) of preliminary research findings presented in conference proceedings are not considered prior publications" [37].

What Are Medical Journals Doing About Plagiarism?

Today when you submit a paper for publication in a refereed journal, the odds are that before it enters the review process, the manuscript will be screened for plagiarism. A common method is the use of "CrossCheck Powered by iThenticate." A favorite of major medical publishers, the CrossCheck service involves "thousands of journals sharing published works with the iThenticate database" [38].

In 2011, Kleinert, writing on behalf of all *Lancet* journals, announced their intention to use CrossCheck to screen not only reports of original research but also all "Seminars, Series, Reviews, and other non-research material that we are interested in publishing" [39].

Even without the use of CrossCheck, it is remarkably easy to check for plagiarism. Try this sort of exercise as a test, as I did: In my 2008 book *White Coat Tales*, there is a chapter titled "Famous Persons as Patients" that begins with the sentence "Health problems don't affect only so-called ordinary people; famous persons suffer illness, get hurt, occasionally experience physical or psychiatric impairment, and eventually breathe their last, just like the rest of us" [40]. I typed in the Google search box the first 12 words of this unremarkable sentence, one that I had picked more or less at random, with no mention of my name or the book title. I then tapped "Return." The first two sites displayed in response to my search were both my *White Coat Tales* book.

How Aware Are Professional Medical Writers and Their Employers of Publication Guidelines?

Given the issues regarding publication of industry-sponsored research in peer-reviewed journals discussed in Chap. 5, it might seem logical to ask if professional medical writers working in the pharmaceutical and medical device industry are aware of guidelines regarding ethical publication practices.

As it turns out, medical writers who are employed to help prepare industry-sponsored research reports for publication know of and apply standard guidelines. This is the conclusion reached by Wager et al. following a survey of 469 professional medical writers, including those working in pharmaceutical or device companies, communication agencies, contract research organizations, or as freelancers. The investigators found that more than 90 % of respondents "routinely refer to Good Publication Practice (GPP2) and the International Committee of Medical Journal Editors' Uniform Requirements." More than three-quarters of respondents told of receiving mandatory training on ethical publication practices [41].

There are some questions to be raised about the publication of industry-sponsored research; think of publication decisions influenced by the prospect of reprint purchases or editorials that read like "advertorials," discussed in Chap. 5. However, the implication that I draw from the Wager et al. study is that the culprits are not the professional medical writers working to make research reports more precise and readable.

What Constitutes Conflict of Interest, Both Intellectual and Financial?

Intellectual conflict of interest occurs when someone brings a bias to the table in a setting—such as a consensus guideline panel—where objectivity is needed to achieve the best outcome. Bion reviewed 6803 publications on the subject of conflict of interest or competing interests. Many described competing interests in the context of published clinical guidelines. The author concludes: "Conflicts of interest (competing interests) and bias are ubiquitous. In medicine, they may have the potential to cause harm to patients or obstruct research and new treatments" [42].

In the setting of research reports published in the literature, financial conflicts of interests are more likely to be found than intellectual conflicts, and are the ones most often reported. Although professional medical writers are unlikely to have financial conflicts of interest, those who conduct clinical research often have relationships with pharmaceutical or medical device companies.

At the University of Pennsylvania in Philadelphia, a 19-year-old subject died in a gene transfer study. It turned out that both the university and the primary investigator were shareholders in a company involved in the study and that the PI and dean of the medical school held patents on the processes involved in the research. This seems an egregious example of conflict of interest in biomedical research [43].

Financial conflict of interest can be an issue in many ways, chiefly when one or more investigators—or their family members—have monetary dealings with pharmaceutical firms funding studies. This can be a little murky since, for example, a 2007 study showed that nearly 60 % of medical school department heads had "personal relationships with industry" [43].

Medical journals and even organizers of continuing medical education programs today are highly sensitive to the need to report all possible financial conflicts of interest. For example, the *Annals of Internal Medicine* requires conflict of interest disclosures by not only all article authors, but also members of panels that help formulate consensus or guideline recommendations, even if those contributors are not named authors on the consensus or guideline statement [44]. Many journals request that authors use the ICMJE conflict of interest form, which is available from the website http://www.icmje.org/conflicts-of-interest/.

We who write for scholarly journals or, for that matter, speak on CME programs, need to do everything we reasonably can to avoid even the appearance of intellectual or financial conflict of interest. As for me, I have carefully avoided buying stock in any pharmaceutical company, not because I consider them to be poor investments, but because I do public speaking, consulting, and peer reviewing, and I do not want to have any suggestion of conflict of interest.

Is There Such a Thing as a Writing Assignment That Skirts the Law?

Yes, there can be. Bauman describes one such scenario. A medical writer is sent to a conference to hear a physician describe a new, but unapproved, use of a drug. Then the medical writer composes a piece about what was heard and his or her employer publishes it in the trade press. This is a way the pharmaceutical industry has found to circumvent US FDA regulations regarding the unapproved use of drugs, and is a violation of ethics, if not the law [45].

References

1. Davidoff F. CSE Task Force on Authorship. Who's the author? Problems with biomedical authorship, and some possible solutions. Sci Editor. 2000;23:111.
2. Wislar JS, et al. Honorary and ghost authorship in high impact biomedical journals: a cross sectional survey. BMJ. 2011;343:d6128.
3. Slone RM. Coauthor's contributions to major papers published in the AJR: frequency of unde-served coauthorship. Am J Roentgenol. 1996;167:571.
4. Koushan M. Ethical considerations in publishing medical articles in Iranian journals. Sci J Fac Med Nis. 2014;31:105.
5. Logdberg L. Being the ghost in the machine: a medical ghostwriter's personal view. PLoS Med. 2011;8(8), e1001071. doi:10.1371/journal.pmed.1001071.
6. Fugh-Berman AJ. The haunting of medical journals: how ghostwriting sold "HRT". PLoS Med. 2010;7(9), e1000335. doi:10.1371/journal.pmed.1000335.
7. PLoS Medicine Editors. Ghostwriting: the dirty little secret of medical publishing that just got bigger. PLoS Med. 2009;6, e1000156. doi:10.1371/journal.pmed.1000156.
8. Jacobs A, et al. European Medical Writers Association (EMWA) guidelines on the role of medical writers in developing peer-reviewed publications. Curr Med Res Opin. 2005;21:317. Available at: http://www.emwa.org/Mum/EMWAguidelines.pdf.
9. International Committee of Medical Journal Editors (ICMJE). Recommendations for the conduct, reporting, editing, and publication of scholarly work in medical journals: sample references. US National Library of Medicine. Available at: http://www.nlm.nih.gov/bsd/uniform_requirements. html.
10. Ilakovac V, et al. Reliability of disclosure forms of authors' contributions. Can Med J. 2007;176:41.
11. Izurieta HS, Thadani N (co-lead-authors), et al. Comparative effectiveness of high-dose versus standard-dose influenza vaccines in US residents aged 65 years and older from 2012 to 2013 using Medicare data: a retrospective cohort analysis. The Lancet Infectious Diseases Online, 2015. doi:10.1016/S1473-3099(14)71087-4. Available at: http://www.thelancet.com/journals/laninf/article/PIIS1473-3099(14)71087-4/abstract.
12. Dudas J. A copyright refresher. United States Patent and Trademark Office. Available from: http://www.uspto.gov/web/offices/dcom/olia/copyright/copyrightrefresher.htm.
13. U.S. Copyright Office. Copyright basics (Circular 1). Available at: http://www.copyright.gov/circs/circ01.pdf.
14. KeytLaw: Fair use: Available at: http://www.keytlaw.com/Copyrights/fairuse.html.
15. Berner ES. Publications in academic medical centers: technology-facilitated culture clash. Acad Med. 2010;89:1.
16. Howard J. Long-awaited ruling in copyright case mostly favors Georgia State U. Chron. High Ed., 13 May 2012. Available at: http://chronicle.com/article/Long-Awaited-Ruling-in/131859/.
17. Onwuegbuzie AJ et al. Bibliographic errors in articles submitted to scholarly journals: the case for research in the schools. Available at: http://www.unco.edu/ae-extra/2006/12/Jiao.html.
18. de Lacey G, et al. How accurate are quotations and references in medical journals? BMJ. 1985;291(6499):884.
19. Ebrahim S, et al. Reanalyses of randomized clinical trial data. JAMA. 2015;312:1024.
20. Rising tide of plagiarism and misconduct in medical research: 2013 iThenticate paper. Available from: http://cdn2.hubspot.net/hub/92785/file-16016700-pdf/docs/ith-medical-plagiarism.pdf/.
21. Roig M. Avoiding plagiarism, self-plagiarism, and other questionable writing practices: a guide to ethical writing. Available from: http://www.cse.msu.edu/~alexliu/plagiarism.pdf.
22. Gould SJ. Ontogeny and phylogeny. Cambridge, MA: Harvard University Press; 1977. p. 35.
23. Benjamin Rush Painting by Peale 1783. This work is in the public domain. Available at: http://commons.wikimedia.org/wiki/File:Benjamin_Rush_Painting_by_Peale_1783.jpg.
24. Ambrose CT. Plagiarism of ideas: Benjamin Rush and Charles Caldwell—a student-mentor dispute. The Pharos. 2014; winter, 15.

25. Marshall E. Two former grad students sue over alleged misuse of ideas. Science. 1999;284:562.
26. Maya Angelou. How I write. The Daily Beast. Available at: http://www.thedailybeast.com/articles/2013/04/10/maya-angelou-how-i-write.html.
27. Das N, et al. Plagiarism: why is it such a big issue for medical writers? Prospect Clin Res. 2011;2:67.
28. Asimov J, Asimov I. How to enjoy writing: a book of aid and comfort. New York: Walker; 1987. p. 51.
29. Asimov I. I. Asimov: a memoir. New York: Doubleday; 1994. p. 205.
30. Roig M. Avoiding plagiarism, self-plagiarism, and other questionable writing practices: a guide to ethical writing. Available from: http://www.cse.msu.edu/~alexliu/plagiarism.pdf/.
31. Holmes profile with signature.jpg. This media file is in the public domain. Available at: http://commons.wikimedia.org/wiki/File:Holmes_profile_with_signature.jpg.
32. Holmes OW. Report of the Committee on Medical Literature. In: Brieger GH, editor. Medical America in the nineteenth century: readings from the literature. Baltimore: Johns Hopkins Press; 1972. p. 45–54.
33. Kravitz RL, et al. From the editors' desk: self-plagiarism and other editorial crimes and misdemeanors. J Gen Intern Med. 2011;26:1.
34. Meta-analysis and the problem of duplicate publication and plagiarism. Scholarly open access: critical analysis of scholarly open-access publishing. Available at: http://scholarlyoa.com/2014/07/29/meta-analyses-and-the-problems-of-duplicate-publication-and-plagiarism/.
35. Choi WS, et al. Duplicate publication of articles used in meta-analyses in Korea. Springerplus. 2014;3:182.
36. Déjà vu: a database of highly similar citations. Virginia Bioinformatics Institute. Available at: http://dejavu.vbi.vt.edu/dejavu/.
37. Academic Medicine: instructions for authors. Available at: http://journals.lww.com/academic-medicine/Pages/InstructionsforAuthors.aspx#prioranduplicatepublication/.
38. CrossCheck Powered by iThenticate. Available at: http://www.ithenticate.com/products/crosscheck/.
39. Kleinert S. Checking for plagiarism, duplicate publication, and text recycling. Lancet. 2011;377:281.
40. Taylor RB. White coat tales: medicine's heroes, heritage, and misadventures. New York: Springer; 2008.
41. Wager E, et al. Medical publishing and peer review: awareness and enforcement of guidelines for publishing industry-sponsored medical research among publication professionals: the Global Publication Survey. BMJ Open. 2014;4, e004780. doi:10.1136/bmjopen-2013-004780.
42. Bion J. Financial and intellectual conflicts of interest: confusion and clarity. Curr Opin Crit Care. 2009;15:583.
43. Johnston J. Conflict of interest in biomedical research. The Hastings Center. Available from: http://www.thehastingscenter.org/Publications/BriefingBook/Detail.aspx?id=2156.
44. Information for authors. Ann Intern Med. Available at: http://annals.org/public/authorsinfo.aspx.
45. Bauman N. Jobs on this list: ethical issues. Available from: http://www.nasw.org/users/nbauman/neuront.htm.

Chapter 7
Remarkable Medical Writing

This chapter is about noteworthy medical writing—and writers. What you read next may not improve your mastery of article structure, grammar, and syntax, but it will offer some examples of outstandingly good and outrageously bad writing, both non-medical and medical. Some of this short chapter is intended to be amusing, perhaps to be enjoyed when you seem bogged down in your own composition. Other sections that follow may provide either tips or warnings that can make you more aware of what to do and not to do in your writing.

Have Some Medical Writers Received the Pulitzer Prize?

The Pulitzer Prize was established in 1917, funded by a bequest from American Publisher Joseph Pulitzer, and is now administered by Columbia University.

There are Pulitzer Prizes awarded in a number of categories, including journalism categories such as "beat reporting," "commentary," "investigative reporting," and "feature writing." There are also awards for "general nonfiction," "fiction," and "history" [1]. In my research, I found several Pulitzer Prizes awarded to journalists writing on medical topics in the "beat reporting" and "feature writing" categories. For example, in 2003 Diana K. Sugg of the *Baltimore Post* won a Pulitzer Prize for "her absorbing, often poignant stories that illuminated complex medical issues through the lives of people" [2].

There is no Pulitzer category specifically for "medical writing," and so it is noteworthy when a medical writer, especially a physician-author writing on a medical topic, is so honored. Here are a few examples; Harvey Cushing (see Fig. 7.1) won a Pulitzer Prize in 1926 for his biography titled *Life of Sir William Osler*. A 1973 Pulitzer Prize went to Robert Coles for *Children of Crisis: A Study of Courage and Fear*. A more recent medical writer recipient of a Pulitzer Prize is Indian-born American physician Siddhartha Mukherjee, who received the prize for his 2010 book *The Emperor of All Maladies: A Biography of Cancer*. Dr. Mukherjee is a

© Springer International Publishing Switzerland 2015
R.B. Taylor, *What Every Medical Writer Needs to Know*,
DOI 10.1007/978-3-319-20264-8_7

Fig. 7.1 American
neurosurgeon and author
Harvey W. Cushing [3]

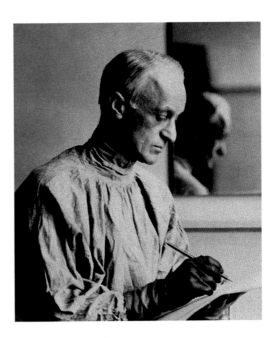

hematologist/oncologist on the faculty of Columbia University. The publisher's note describes his book as "a magnificent, profoundly humane 'biography' of cancer—from its first documented appearances thousands of years ago through the epic battles in the twentieth century to cure, control, and conquer it to a radical new understanding of its essence" [4].

Have Medical Writers Been Recipients of Other Writing Awards?

A few physicians have been recipients of the National Book Award. Physician Victor G. Heiser received the 1936 nonfiction award for his autobiography titled *An American Doctor's Odyssey: Adventures in Forty-Five Countries*, describing his work to combat typhoid, cholera, smallpox, and leprosy. In 1950 William Carlos Williams was the awardee in the Poetry category for *Paterson: Book III and Selected Poems*.

Robert Coles received a Pulitzer Prize for General Non-Fiction in 1973 for his series of books *Children of Crisis*. Lewis Thomas wrote a series of essays in the *New England Journal of Medicine* (NEJM), and a collection of those essays, *The Lives of a Cell: Notes of a Biology Watcher* (1974), won the author 1975 National Book Awards in two categories, Arts and Letters and The Sciences (both awards were split). Thomas also won a Christopher Award for his book.

Subsequently, *The Medusa and the Snail*, another Lewis Thomas collection of NEJM essays, also earned the National Book Award in Science. American surgeon Sherwin B. Nuland received the award in 1994 for his work *How We Die*, about the controversy surrounding physician-assisted suicide.

As to the Nobel Prize in Literature, I found that Laureates included authors Winston Churchill, Nadine Gordimer, Saul Bellow, and Aleksandr Solzhenitsyn, but I could not identify a single medical writer.

I also scanned the winners of the American Book Award, Neustadt International Prize for Literature, and the Man Booker International Prize for Literature, but could not spot a medical writer among the many winners, at least one whose name I recognized.

What About Awards to Recognize Remarkable Achievements in Medical Writing?

The American Medical Writers Association (AMWA) sponsors awards each year recognizing exceptional books intended for readers in three categories: physicians, non-physician health care professionals, and the public/health care consumers. Here are the 2014 winners:

Books for Physicians: Miguel A. Cubano, for *Emergency War Surgery, 4th United States Revision*.

Books for Non-physician Health Care Professionals: Kenneth R. Ginsburg and Sara B. Kinsman, for *Reaching Teens: Strength-Based Communications to Build Resilience and Support Healthy Adolescent Development*.

Books for Public or Health Care Consumers: Sheri Fink, for *Five Days at Memorial: Life and Death in a Storm-Ravaged Hospital*.

AMWA also sponsors other awards. One is the annual Eric W. Martin Award for Excellence in Medical Writing, named for a past president of AMWA. There are two award categories—professional audience articles and public or health care consumer articles.

The AMWA John P. McGovern Award honors a noteworthy contribution to any of the various modes of medical communication. The award bears the name of the founder of the McGovern Allergy Clinic in Houston, Texas and the co-founder of the American Osler Society. The 2014 award recipient was Gary Schwitzer, adjunct associate professor at the University of Minnesota School of Public Health and publisher of *HealthNewsReview.org*.

The AMWA Walter C. Alvarez Award recognizes excellence in communicating health care developments and concepts to the public. Physician-author Alvarez wrote a number of books for the lay audience and penned a regular syndicated medical column widely published in newspapers. His name is eponymously memorialized as the Alvarez syndrome, describing a condition of abdominal bloating in the absence of gas in the intestinal tract.

The 2014 Alvarez Award went to Rosemary Gibson, an editor for *JAMA Internal Medicine* and senior advisor to the Hastings Center. Gibson's latest book is *Medicare Meltdown: How Wall Street and Washington Are Ruining Medicare and How to Fix It* (New York: Rowman & Littlefield; 2013).

What Might Be Some Tongue-in-Cheek Special Awards in Biomedical Writing?

Alert: In the Introduction to this chapter, I foretold some items intended to be amusing. What you will read next is whimsical—not to be taken too seriously. That is, unless some of your writing might be in contention for one of the following awards.

Along with works meriting the Pulitzer Prize, National Book Award, Nobel Prize in Literature, the following achievements also deserve recognition. In several instances, I serve as the sole judge as to honored recipients, but I welcome nominations for the next round of awards.

The Most Authors on a Scientific Article

For 2011, the latest year for which results are available, the award must be considered a tie. According to *ScienceWatch*, in this year 140 scientific papers listed more than 1000 authors. An early record was achieved a few years ago when a paper discussing the effect of pravastatin, published in *Circulation*, had more than 2400 authors. We have since seen physics papers with more than 3000 authors [5]. To borrow an "authorism" attributed to Indiana University information scientist Blaise Cronin, we are seeing continuing growth in "hyperauthorship" [6].

The Most Intriguing Title(s)

Because there are various models of medical writing, there are subcategories of the Most Intriguing Title Award: lecture, op-ed, scholarly article, and book.

- **Best lecture title award**: *Give Canary Another Seed: Part Two*. I encountered this lecture title more than three decades ago shortly after joining the faculty at Bowman Gray School of Medicine, now the Wake Forest University School of Medicine. I didn't know then and don't know now what the lecture was about, but the title was intriguing, and—as we can see—memorable. I wonder what was covered in Part One.
- **Best op-ed title award**: *Ghost Writers in the Sky*. (No authors listed. J Urol. 2008;179:809.) Being that this is a book about medical writing, I could not

ignore this title. First runner-up: *The Disease of the Little Paper*, describing the patient with a long list of problems. (Koven S. N Engl J Med. 2014;371:2251.)

- **Most colorful title of a scholarly article**: The winner is *Not Guppies, Nor Goldfish, But Tumble Dryers, Noriega, Jesse Jackson, Panties, Car Crashes, Bird Books, and Stevie Wonder* [Storms G et al. Memory and Cognition. 1998:26:143]. This article is all of three pages long, making the title almost as long as the text.

- First runner-up for the Most Colorful Title Award: *The Bugs Eat the Waste: What Else Is There to Know? Changing Professional Hegemony in the Design of Sewage Treatment Plants.* [Van de Poel I. Soc Stud Sci. 2008;38:605.] Was this a scientific paper? Maybe, or maybe not. But it certainly had a catchy title.

- **Most imaginative article subtitle**: Subtitles are explanatory phrases, intended to clarify a somewhat vague title or to appeal to the reader's interests. For example, a scholarly subtitle for an article titled: *Comparison of Drugs A and B in the Treatment of Hyperlipidemia* might be *A Randomized, Controlled Study*. Medical authors have recently been searching for witty subtitles. Here is a winner and a runner-up:

Hepatitis C Treatment: Stuck Between a Rock and a Hard Place But Hoping to Be Rescued Soon. [Katz MH. JAMA Int Med. 2014;174:212.] Let's hope that the paper identifies a rescuer.

Practice-Based Research: Blue Highways on the NIH Roadmap. (Westfall JM et al. JAMA. 2007;297:403.) The allusion is to old highway maps that depicted main roads as red and back roads as blue. Practice-based research thrives in rural practice settings, aspiring to use community practices to answer clinical questions raised by actual practicing physicians.

- **Most imaginative book title**: My vote goes to *The Man Who Mistook His Wife for a Hat: and Other Clinical Tales*, by Oliver Sacks (see Fig. 7.2). [Sacks O. New York: Touchstone; 1998.] Also the author of *An Anthropologist on Mars* and *Awakenings*, physician-author Olivier Sacks describes uncommon manifestations of various neurologic disorders.

The Most Arcane Use of Medical Jargon Likely to Send Me to the Dictionary

Consider the following published abstract [8]:

"Goodpasture's disease, or anti-glomerular basement membrane (anti-GBM) disease, is a systemic autoimmune disorder defined by anti-GBM antibody-mediated damage (mainly immunoglobulin G-1) resulting in progressive crescentic glomerulonephritis and, frequently, diffuse pulmonary alveolar hemorrhage. It may be regarded as a "conformeropathy" where the quaternary structure of the $\alpha345NC1$ hexamer that constitutes GBM undergoes a conformational change, exposing pathogenic epitopes on the $\alpha3$ and $\alpha5$ chains, eliciting a pathogenic autoantibody anti-GBM response."

I cannot find "conformeropathy" in any of my medical dictionaries.

Fig. 7.2 Oliver Sacks,
American physician and
author, 2009. Photo credit:
Erik Charlton [7]

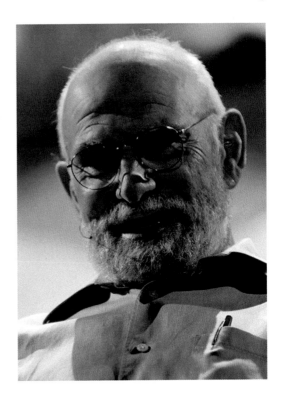

Heaviest Medical Reference Book in Single Volume

Until superseded by a weightier challenger, I claim one of my own edited books as
holding this dubious distinction. The second edition of my edited reference book
Family Medicine: Principles and Practice, published in 1983 and with 2020 pages
on good-quality paper, weighs 12 lb on my bathroom scale [9]. I am not proud of
this. It really should have been much trimmer, or else published in two volumes.
A book of this heft represents literary macrosomia by any definition. The book,
intended to be the same reasonable 1200-page length as the first edition, just seemed
to grow as one author after another vastly exceeded page allocations. More than
three decades ago, I was an inexperienced book editor working with a young
"sponsoring editor" who loved the project too much. She encouraged me, "If it is
important, don't cut it." As a result, the book became huge, and publishing as one
volume instead of two was just one more mistake.

The huge size of the book almost caused its demise. But Springer went on to
support a subsequent edition and, today, we are preparing the seventh edition of
Family Medicine: Principles and Practice, with strict attention to page allocations
for contributing authors.

Are There Some Humorous Awards for Bad Writing?

In addition to some awards for scientific writing, my research revealed three contests with awards for outrageously bad writing for the public. I am sad to report that only two of them survive today.

The Bulwer-Lytton Fiction Contest

In the year 1830, Victorian author Lord Edward Bulwer-Lytton secured a permanent place in the history of English literature as he began his novel titled *Paul Clifford* with the now-famous sentence that begins, "It was a dark and stormy night" [10] (see Fig. 7.3).

Few today recall that Bulwer-Lytton also gave us the aphorism "the pen is mightier than the sword" and the phrases "the almighty dollar" and "the great unwashed." No, we remember him for his single opening line, popularized a few years ago as Snoopy in the *Peanuts* comic strip aspired to be a writer in spite of repeated rejections. The Baron is eponymously memorialized in the annual Bulwer-Lytton Fiction Contest begun in 1962 by Professor Scott Rice at San Jose State University in California.

The rules of the contest are simple. Each entrant must submit a single sentence. By tradition, most entries are opening lines of nonexistent novels [12]. Each year the contest attracts thousands of entries from the USA and abroad. Although there are special awards in categories such as Romance, Fantasy, Adventure, Crime, and others, there is no category for medical or scientific writing. It is of course a "fiction" contest.

Fig. 7.3 English novelist and politician Edward Bulwer-Lytton, 1st Baron Lytton [11]

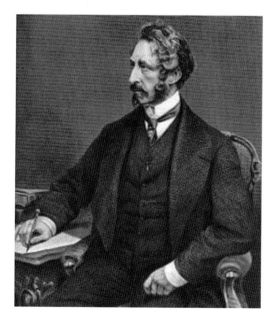

The 2014 winner of the Bulwer-Lytton Fiction Contest was Elizabeth Dorfman of Bainbridge Island, Washington, who penned [12]:

> When the dead moose floated into view the famished crew cheered—this had to mean land!—but Captain Walgrove, flinty-eyed and clear headed thanks to the starvation cleanse in progress, gave fateful orders to remain on the original course and await the appearance of a second and confirming moose.

But as writers, perhaps we should examine the words that have earned Bulwer-Lytton perpetual derision. The phrase "It was a dark and stormy night" seems, to me, unremarkable. It is short and precise. Only one word has more than one syllable. It uses old, strong words. Today the phrase is a cliché, but in 1830 it was a freshly penned thought. But, as Paul Harvey used to say, here is the rest of the story—the full sentence that began the book *Paul Clifford* [10]:

> It was a dark and stormy night; the rain fell in torrents, except at occasional intervals, when it was checked by a violent gust of wind which swept up the streets (for it is in London that our scene lies), rattling along the housetops, and fiercely agitating the scanty flame of the lamps that struggled against the darkness.

Given the florid prose characteristic of the early 1800s writing, is the sentence really so bad? Yes, it is somewhat long and rambling. And the author likes adjectives and adverbs such as violent, fiercely, and scanty. But the verb forms are vigorous and I can follow what the author is saying without having to reread the sentence several times. If submitted today to the Bulwer-Lytton Fiction Contest, would this entry even make the first round of cuts?

The Bad Sex in Fiction Award

Since 1993 the *Literary Review*, published in London, has sponsored an annual "Bad Sex in Fiction Award." Several of the entries I found were too lurid for this book. The 2013 award winner for Bad Sex in Fiction was *The City of Devi* penned by Manil Suri, a novel set in Mumbai, India, when the city is under threat of a nuclear bomb [13]. The winning prose, although somewhat inscrutable as a "sex" scene, is suitable for mixed company [14]:

> Surely supernovas explode that instant, somewhere, in some galaxy. The hut vanishes, and with it the sea and the sands—only Karun's body, locked with mine, remains. We streak like superheroes past suns and solar systems, we dive through shoals of quarks and atomic nuclei. In celebration of our breakthrough fourth star, statisticians the world over rejoice.

The Philosophy and Literature *Bad Writing Contest*

From 1995 to 1998 the journal *Philosophy and Literature*, published by the Johns Hopkins University Press, sponsored the "Bad Writing Contest" [15]. It might well have been called the "Most Murky Prose Contest." Here, penned by Professor Judith Butler, is the winning submission for the final year of the contest [16].

The move from a structuralist account in which capital is understood to structure social relations in relatively homologous ways to a view of hegemony in which power relations are subject to repetition, convergence, and rearticulation brought the question of temporality into the thinking of structure, and marked a shift from a form of Althusserian theory that takes structural totalities as theoretical objects to one in which the insights into the contingent possibility of structure inaugurate a renewed conception of hegemony as bound up with the contingent sites and strategies of the rearticulation of power.

This paragraph is actually one long sentence, and it lost me in the third line. Like other meritorious Bad Writing Contest entries cited, it is so amusingly impenetrable that it makes me wish the contest still existed. Nevertheless, as I typed this page, my MS Word spelling and grammar checker highlighted three words—structuralist, rearticulation, and Althusserian—but happily accepted the structure of the sentence.

What Are Some of the Most Unnecessary and Ridiculous Articles in the Scientific Literature, Reporting Studies We Taxpayers Probably Supported?

Sometimes we must wonder about who spends their career studying the sort of questions addressed in the articles below. And who in the world funds them? Consider the following:

- **Effects of cocaine on honeybee dance behavior**: Here's the background: It seems that honeybees dance to tell nest mates about floral resources they have detected. The researchers found: "Treatment with a low dose of cocaine increased the likelihood and rate of bees dancing after foraging but did not otherwise increase locomotor activity. This is consistent with cocaine causing forager bees to overestimate the value of the floral resources they collected" [17]. So maybe if we give bees cocaine they will produce more honey, or less? And will the honey be laced with cocaine?
- **The "booty call": a compromise between men's and women's ideal mating strategies**: The compromise seems to be "between men's and women's ideal mating strategies that allows men greater sexual access and women an ongoing opportunity to evaluate potential long-term mates" [18]. Is this what scientists call dating today?
- **Alcohol consumption and the intention to engage in unprotected sex**: The study conclusion: Alcohol consumption increases the risk of unprotected sex [19]. I, for one, am shocked! On a methodologic note, one might fantasize about how to conduct this study, until noticing that it was a meta-analysis of previously published literature.
- **Salmonella excretion in joy-riding pigs**: The Oregon State Health Division and the Liverpool School of Tropical Medicine collaborated on this groundbreaking study [20].

And, not to be outdone:

- **The nature of navel fluff**: In reading this article, I learned that "Old T-shirts or dress shirts produce less naval fuzz than brand new T-shirts" [21]. Somehow, I am sure, this advances our treasury of scientific knowledge. As for me, I now know why I resist discarding my old T-shirts. Too much fluff in the new ones.

All of these studies are memorialized in PubMed so that they can be accessed by researchers with similar interests.

What Are Some of the Most Intriguing First Sentences in the Medical Literature?

As all writers know, the first sentence in an article or chapter is probably the most important. If the reader is not captured by this sentence, sometimes called the "hook," he or she may not go on to the brilliant prose that follows. In a scientific article, the opening sentence in the Abstract or Introduction is typically a general statement setting the stage for more specific facts to follow. Consider these actual first sentences.

"Sword swallowers know their occupation is dangerous." A survey of 46 members of the Sword Swallowers Association International revealed, among other facts, that sore throats (aka "sword throats") were common when learning the craft [22].

"The purpose of this study was to investigate the significance of wet underwear and to compare any influence of fiber-type material and textile construction of underwear on thermoregulatory responses and thermal comfort of humans during rest in the cold" [23]. The authors of the study concluded that, in cold weather, wet underwear resulted in a "significant cooling effect." I suspect the researchers' mothers could have told them about the hazards of wearing wet underwear in cold weather. This study was not a contender for the Nobel Prize that year.

"Waist circumference is a simple and valuable anthropometric measure of total and intra-abdominal body fat" [24]. Belt size is an "anthropometric measure." And abdominal girth can indicate the amount of body fat. Astounding! Who would have guessed?

What Seems to Be the Most Down-to-Earth and Comprehensible Medical Journal?

My vote for the most reader-friendly medical journal goes to the *British Medical Journal* (BMJ). Not only is the editing superior to most other journals, but also the BMJ has the courage to publish studies that other journals would reject out of hand. One such report is the paper titled "Sword Swallowing and Its Side Effects," described above.

For years the Christmas issue of BMJ has featured reports that relate to the holiday. In 2012 we find "Why Rudolph's Nose is Red: An Observational Study."

The researchers report: "The nasal microcirculation of reindeer is richly vascularized, with a vascular density 25 % higher than in humans. These results highlight the intrinsic physiological properties of Rudolph's legendary luminous red nose, which help to protect it from freezing during sleigh rides and to regulate the temperature of the reindeer's brain, factors essential for flying reindeer pulling Santa Claus's sleigh under extreme temperatures" [25].

In September 2014 the Journal published a study involving more than 200,000 women, examining a possible relationship between skirt size change (as a proxy for weight change) and postmenopausal breast cancer, confirming that increased skirt size, indicating an increase in body fat, increases the risk of breast cancer [26].

This was a well-designed study that, nevertheless, provoked at least one feminist critic who, writing in my local newspaper, described the report as "patronizing and paternalistic" [27].

My all-time favorite is the British Medical Journal (BMJ) report by Palazzo et al. titled "Surgeons Swear When Operating: Fact Or Myth?" In fact, improbable as it may seem, surgeons do curse in the operating room. And what specialists are the prime offenders? Orthopedic surgeons swear most of all [28].

And so, yes, there is a place for humor in scholarly biomedical journals.

What May Be the Most Recognized Medical Book in All of Medicine?

In a *Journal of the American Medical Association* (JAMA) review of the 18th edition of *Harrison's Principles of Internal Medicine*, Preeti N. Malani describes the new edition as "a worthy update to what is arguably the most recognized book in all of medicine." Malani points out that the first edition was compiled 63 years ago and he highlights the many changes that must be incorporated in each new edition [29].

Is There One Most Engaging, Readable, and Yet Erudite Medical Book Available Today?

Your answer to this question will depend on your age and specialty. My personal favorite is Sapira's *Art and Science of Bedside Diagnosis*, originally published in 1990, and now in its fourth edition, currently edited by Jane M. Orient [30].

Sapira began the Preface to the first edition with a quotation from Wieger's book on the history of Chinese characters [31], citing the perils of false teaching and learning:

> As the decay of the Chou Dynasty grew worse, studies were neglected and the scribes became more and more ignorant. When they did not remember the genuine characters, they blunderingly invented a false one. These non-genuine characters, copied out again by other ignorant writers, became usual.

This somewhat unlikely introduction is followed by Sapira's clear statement of his intent in writing the book: "The goal of this book is to help the reader achieve the correct personal, metaphysical, and epistemologic perspectives on the artful science of the clinical examination. This is not a textbook of medicine …" [30].

The things I like about Sapira's book are several: He gives insights into why we do what we do in physician diagnosis, in some cases showing the truth of the quotation regarding incorrect Chinese characters. On page 297, he writes that "the custom of having the patient say "99" during the palpation of the chest arose from a misunderstanding of our medical ancestors, who during a postgraduate year in Germany observed patients being told to say "99" in German (i.e., *neun und nunzig*, the "eu" diphthong being pronounced as in our words "boy" or "toy"). The direct translation into English eliminates the diphthong and changes the spectral characteristic of the sound so that less energy is expressed below 80 Hz. (If the German speakers had wanted our "nine" sound, they would have asked the patient to say "*nein*" (no).) To best approximate the German, we should use the words "boy" or "toy." This misunderstanding has been perpetuated in textbooks for generations.

Some of his anatomical figures are actually based on photographs of famous statues, such as Fig. 14.3, on page 276, showing a Satyr with a goiter in a statue by Michelangelo.

Finally, he offers unexpected literary allusions, such as beginning Chapter 6 (page 101) on the vital signs. Here we find a quotation from Ernest Hemingway's *Death in the Afternoon* [32]:

> At this point it is necessary that you see a bullfight. If I were to describe one it would not be the one that you would see, since the bullfighters and the bulls are all different, and if I were to explain the possible variations as I went along the chapter would be interminable …

I think that Sapira's point in telling about a bullfight echoes the Oslerism: "To study the phenomena of disease without books is to sail an uncharted sea, while to study books without patients is not to go to sea at all" [33].

Several decades ago, an unsympathetic reviewer stated that one of my (early) authored books was a good example of the fact that medicine is now so complex that we should no longer have single-author books. I think that Sapira's *Art and Science of Bedside Diagnosis* belies that opinion.

Is There a Single Most Influential Bioscientific Paper of All Time?

My choice for the most impactful medical writing of all time goes to Edward Jenner, author of "An Inquiry into the Causes and Effects of the Variolae Vaccine, or Cowpox," published in 1798 [34]. In Jenner's time, smallpox was a major cause of death in Europe, killing some 60 million people in Europe during the seventeenth century (see Fig. 7.4). Those who survived were typically scarred for life [36, 37].

Fig. 7.4 Child with smallpox in Bangladesh, 1973. Photo credit: CDC/ James Hicks [35]

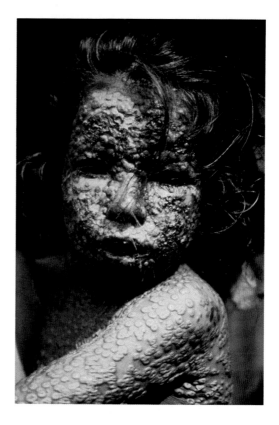

Smallpox, although officially declared "eradicated" in 1980, still remains incurable. From 1798 until the date the final infected patient was discovered in Somalia, Jenner's discovery that a mild infection with cowpox could reliably prevent small-pox saved millions of lives. I don't think the findings reported in any other medical report equal this achievement.

What Was the Longest Title of a Research Paper Ever Published?

A few years ago a Ph.D. student wrote a script that answered that question, based on characters, not words. Here is what he identified as the longest title of a research paper: "The Nucleotide Sequence Of A 3.2 Kb Segment Of Mitochondrial Maxicircle DNA From *Crithidia Fasciculate* Containing The Gene For Cytochrome Oxidase Subunit III, The N-Terminal Part Of The Apocytochrome *B* Gene And A Possible Frameshift Gene; Further Evidence For The Use Of Unusual Initiator

Triplets In Trypanosome Mitochondria" [38]. The paper was published in the journal *Nucleic Acids Research*, which has a respectable Five-Year Impact Factor of 8.378.

The information is an admittedly a little out of date (1987), and represents an opportunity for an aspiring author to reproduce the study and report it to all of us, perhaps with an even longer title.

What Is the Most Infamous Medical Report of Modern Times?

Without a doubt this is the paper titled "Ileal-Lymphoid Nodular Hyperplasia, Non-Specific Colitis, and Pervasive Developmental Disorder in Children," by Andrew J. Wakefield and twelve (12) hapless coauthors. The paper was published in *The Lancet* in 1998 and subsequently retracted by that journal in 2010. Based on the comments of the parents of 12 children recruited for his study and using data later described as fraudulent, Wakefield postulated a link between the measles-mumps-rubella (MMR) vaccine and childhood developmental disorders, notably autism [39, 40].

It might not have been so bad and Wakefield's paper might have merely been one more bogus report in the literature if not for the influence on parental decisions following the publicity that accompanied the article. Strobe reports: "Immunization rates in Britain dropped from 92 % to 73 %, and were as low as 50 % in some parts of London. The effect was not nearly as dramatic in the United States, but researchers have estimated that as many as 125,000 US children born in the late 1990s did not get the MMR vaccine because of the Wakefield splash" [41]. In fact, the 1998 report has spawned an anti-vaccine movement that persists today, leaving tens of thousands of children susceptible to readily preventable childhood illnesses. Wakefield must share some blame for the 2015 "Disney World" outbreak of measles in the USA.

At least ten of the coauthors have subsequently repudiated the paper. Flaherty has called the article "the most damaging medical hoax of the last 100 years" [42]. As for Dr. Wakefield, his license to practice medicine in the UK has been revoked [43]. And in 2011, Medscape placed him at the top of their list of "Worst Physicians of the Year" [44].

References

1. The Pulitzer Prizes. Available from: http://www.pulitzer.org/.
2. 2003 Pulitzer Prize: journalism awards, beat reporting. Available at: http://en.wikipedia.org/wiki/2003_Pulitzer_Prize/.
3. Harvey Williams Cushing.jpg. Source: http://wellcomeimages.org/indexplus/image/V0026788.html. This file is licensed under the Creative Commons Attribution 4.0 International license. Available at: http://commons.wikimedia.org/wiki/File:Harvey_Williams_Cushing.jpg.

4. The emperor of all maladies: a biography of cancer. Publisher's book description. Available from: http://www.amazon.com/Emperor-All-Maladies-Biography-Cancer/dp/1439170916/ref=la_B003SNL6EA_1_1?s=books&ie=UTF8&qid=1398366065&sr=1-1/.

5. Multiauthored papers: onward and upward: Science-Watch. Available at: http://archive.sciencewatch.com/newsletter/2012/201207/multiauthor_papers/.

6. Cronin B. Hyperauthorship: a postmodern perversion or evidence of a structural shift in scholarly communication practices? J Am Soc Inf Sci Technol. 2001;52:558.

7. Oliver Sacks at TED 2009.jpg. This file is licensed under the Creative Commons Attribution 2.0 Generic license. Available at: http://commons.wikimedia.org/wiki/File:Oliver_Sacks_at_TED_2009.jpg.

8. Chan AL. Cutting edge issues in Goodpasture's syndrome. Clin Rev All Immunol. 2011;41:151.

9. Taylor RB. Family medicine: principles and practice. 2nd ed. New York: Springer; 1983.

10. Bulwer-Lytton E. Paul Clifford. Available at: http://www.readbookonline.net/read/20417/57414/.

11. Edward bulwer-lytton.jpg. This image is in the public domain because its copyright has expired. Available at: http://commons.wikimedia.org/wiki/File:Edward_bulwer-lytton.jpg.

12. The Bulwer-Lytton Fiction Contest. Available at: http://www.bulwer-lytton.com/.

13. Kennedy M. Bad sex award goes to Manil Suri and his shoals of atomic nuclei. The Guardian, 3 Dec 2013. Available at: http://www.theguardian.com/books/2013/dec/03/manil-suri-wins-bad-sex-book-award-city-of-devi/.

14. Suri M. The city of Devi. New York: Norton; 2013.

15. The Bad Writing Contest. Philosophy and literature. Available at: http://denisdutton.com/bad_writing.htm.

16. Butler J. Further reflections on the conversations of our times. Diacritics. 1997;27:13.

17. Barron AB, et al. Effects of cocaine on honeybee dance behavior. J Exp Biol. 2009;212:163.

18. Jonason PK, et al. The "booty call": a compromise between men's and women's ideal mating strategies. J Sex Res. 2009;46:460.

19. Remh J, et al. Alcohol consumption and the intention to engage in unprotected sex: systematic review and meta-analysis of experimental studies. Addiction. 2012;107:1360.

20. Williams LP, et al. Salmonella excretion in joy-riding pigs. Am J Public Health Nations Health. 1970;60:926.

21. Steinhauser G. The nature of navel fluff. Med Hypotheses. 2009;72:623.

22. Whitcombe B. Sword swallowing and its side effects. BMJ. 2006;333:1285.

23. Bakkevig MK, et al. Impact of wet underwear on thermoregulator responses and thermal comfort in the cold. Ergonomics. 1994;8:1375.

24. Ford ES, et al. Trends in mean waist circumference and abdominal obesity among US adults, 1999–2012. JAMA. 2014;312:1151.

25. Ince C, et al. Why Rudolph's nose is red: an observational study. BMJ. 2012;345, e8311.

26. Fourkala EO, et al. Association of skirt size and postmenopausal breast cancer risk in older women: a cohort study within the UK Collaborative Trial of Ovarian Cancer Screening (UKCTOCS). BMJ Open. 2014;4, e005400.

27. Barreca G. Questions you can't skirt past. The Virginian-Pilot, 13 Oct 2014, p. 17.

28. Palazzo FF, et al. Surgeons swear when operating: fact or myth? BMJ. 1999;319:1611.

29. Malani PN. Review of Harrison's principles of internal medicine. JAMA. 2012;308:1813.

30. Orient JM. Sapira's art and science of bedside diagnosis. 3rd ed. Philadelphia, PA: Lippincott, Williams & Wilkins; 2005.

31. Wieger L. Chinese characters. 2nd ed. New York: Dover; 1965.

32. Hemingway E. Death in the afternoon. New York: Scribner; 1932.

33. Sir William Osler quotes, or Oslerisms. Available at: http://lifeinthefastlane.com/resources/oslerisms/.

34. Jenner E. An inquiry into the causes and effects of the variola vaccine, or cowpox. London: Sampson Low; 1798.

35. Child with smallpox Bangladesh edit.jpg. This image is a work of the Centers for Disease Control and Prevention, part of the United States Department of Health and Human Services, taken or made as part of an employee's official duties. As a work for the U.S. Federal government,

Child_with_Smallpox_Bangladesh_edit.jpg.

36. Plotkin SA, et al. Vaccines. Philadelphia, PA: Saunders; 1999.
37. Asimov I. Isaac Asimov's book of facts. New York: Bell; 1979. p. 68.
38. Sloof P, et al. The nucleotide sequence of a 3.2 kb segment of mitochondrial maxicircle DNA
    from *Crithidia fasciculate* containing the gene for cytochrome oxidase subunit III, the
    N-terminal part of the apocytochrome *b* gene and a possible frameshift gene; further evidence
    for the use of unusual initiator triplets in trypanosome mitochondria. Nucleic Acids Res.
    1987;15:51.
39. Wakefield AJ, et al. Ileal-lymphoid nodular hyperplasia, non-specific colitis, and pervasive
    developmental disorder in children. Lancet. 1998;351:637.
40. Godlee F, et al. Wakefield's article linking MMR vaccine and autism was fraudulent. BJM.
    2011;342:c7452.
41. Stobbe M. Will autism fraud report be a vaccine booster? The Boston Globe, Associated Press,
    7 Jan 2011.
42. Flaherty DK. The vaccine-autism connection: a public health crisis caused by unethical medical
    practices and fraudulent science. Ann Pharmacother. 2011;45:1302.
43. Meikie J, et al. MMR row doctor Andrew Wakefield struck off register. London: The Guardian;
    2010.
44. Best and worst physicians of the year. Medscape 2011. Available at: http://www.medscape.
    com/features/slideshow/physicians-of-the-year/2011.

Chapter 8
Backstories of Medical Writers and Writing

In 1751, George Washington, later to become America's first president, traveled to Barbados, where he contracted smallpox [1]. Washington survived the disease, leaving him with facial scars and a lifelong immunity to the disease. Winston Churchill—statesman, orator, and painter—was also a skilled bricklayer, so skilled that in 1928, while he was serving as Chancellor of the Exchequer, he received membership in the Amalgamated Union of Building Trades Workers, the union of masons and bricklayers [2]. In the early 1950s in England, Margaret Roberts supported herself working as a research chemist developing emulsifiers for ice cream. Later, in 1979, and following her marriage to Denis Thatcher, she—now Margaret Thatcher—would become the only woman to serve as Prime Minister of the UK [3].

Our heroes and their works never spring fully formed from nothingness. And their lives sometimes take odd turns. There are always interesting stories—the seldom-told anecdotes behind the often-repeated legends, the odd facts behind the works and their creators. If I were engaged in the information technology industry, for example, I would like to know all about the Bill Gates story and how Steve Jobs and Steve Wosniak began the Apple Inc. in a garage. If I were a poet—a truly difficult way to make a living these days—I would read about the adventures and foibles of the world's great poets: Elizabeth Barrett Browning, William Wordsworth, Walt Whitman, and others. Aspiring novelists should try to get into the minds of F. Scott Fitzgerald and Virginia Woolf. And so, as medical writers we can enrich our lives by learning some little-known tales of memorable medical writers and their works.

© Springer International Publishing Switzerland 2015
R.B. Taylor, *What Every Medical Writer Needs to Know*,
DOI 10.1007/978-3-319-20264-8_8

Who Was the First Known Medical Writer in History, and Why Is He a Remarkable Figure in History?

The first medical writer we can identify was Imhotep, who lived in the twenty-seventh century BCE, and who I mentioned briefly in Chap. 1 (see Fig. 8.1). He is described by Osler as "the first figure of a physician to stand out clearly from the mists of antiquity" [5]. Of course, there are fragments of even earlier medical writings describing disease, many recorded in the cuneiform manner, but the authors remain unknown, and so Imhotep is the first medical author we can identify with reasonable certainty. Some of Imhotep's medical writings, inscribed on papyrus and chiefly describing injuries of various sorts, can be viewed today. The document, called the Edwin Smith papyrus, can be found at the New York Academy of Medicine in New York City.

Imhotep was not only the leading physician of his day. He also held the title of Maker of Vases in Chief and is believed to be the designer of the step pyramid of Djoser at Saqqara. He constructed his own tomb, hiding it so well from tomb raiders that it has never been found [6].

What Was the First Medical Book to Be Printed and What Is Its Serendipitous History?

The first medical book to be printed was *De Medicina*, written by Aulus Cornelius Celsus in Latin in the first century BCE. The book was printed in 1478 in Florence, Italy, by printer Nicolaus Laurentii, who was the first to use copper plate engravings [7]. This came 28 years after the invention of the moveable-type printing press by Johannes Gutenberg in Germany in the year 1450.

Fig. 8.1 Statuette of Imhotep in the Louvre Museum, Paris. Photo credit: Hu Toya [4]

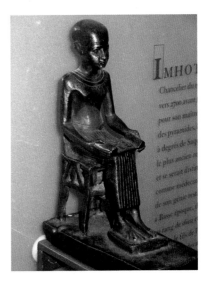

Celsus has been described as an author, editor, and encyclopedist, but he was probably not a physician. He, nevertheless, left us a window into the practice of medicine in ancient Rome. It is fortunate for students of medical history that of all the works of Celsus, what survives is his description of medical practice. The background story of *De Medicina*, at least the part we know today, is that the document was lost sometime around the year 850, during the medieval times when science was subordinated to theology, and was not found again until 1426–1427 [8] (see Fig. 8.2).

What Was the Most-Important-Ever Article in The New England Journal of Medicine and What Is Curious About It?

According to Buckley writing in Now@NEJM, a blog for Physicians about the NEJM, the most important article published in the century-long history of the *New England Journal of Medicine* (NEJM) was "Insensibility during Surgical Operations Produced by Inhalation," by Henry Jacob Bigelow, published on November 18, 1846, in what was then the *Boston Medical and Surgical Journal*. Buckley tells that the choice of this article was based on a vote of the journal's readers as part of the 200th anniversary celebration of the founding of the NEJM. In the voting, the article describing the first reported demonstration of successful inhalation anesthesia eclipsed subsequent articles describing studies on the attenuated measles vaccine, the use of aspirin to prevent heart attacks, and the first treatment of stroke [10]. The article describes the October 16, 1846, surgical removal of a tumor from the neck of a patient under ether anesthesia, leading the surgical theater at Massachusetts General Hospital to be subsequently called the "ether dome."

There are several interesting stories behind the article, which truly describes a turning point in the history of anesthesia and surgery. The first is that, while we all recall dentist William T.G. Morton as the person who administered ether as the successful surgical anesthetic in the demonstration, Morton is not a coauthor on the article. Neither is the surgeon, Doctor James Collins Warren, although both are mentioned in Bigelow's article. Bigelow, the paper's author, was a hospital staff surgeon who arranged the epic event. I submit that this again shows the power of writing. Had he not written his paper describing the occasion, Bigelow would not be remembered as the author of the NEJM's most important article ever [11].

But, wait, there's more! The last page of Bigelow's paper tells that "the patent has been secured." Morton wanted both fame and wealth, even if he did not contribute to the paper describing ether anesthesia's debut. He called his substance "Letheon" and on November 12, 1846, less than a month following his now-legendary demonstration, Morton secured US Patent Number 4848. In the end, efforts to enforce the patent proved "ethereal," and ether came to enjoy wide use among surgeons and dentists, leading the way to today's (usually) painless surgery [12].

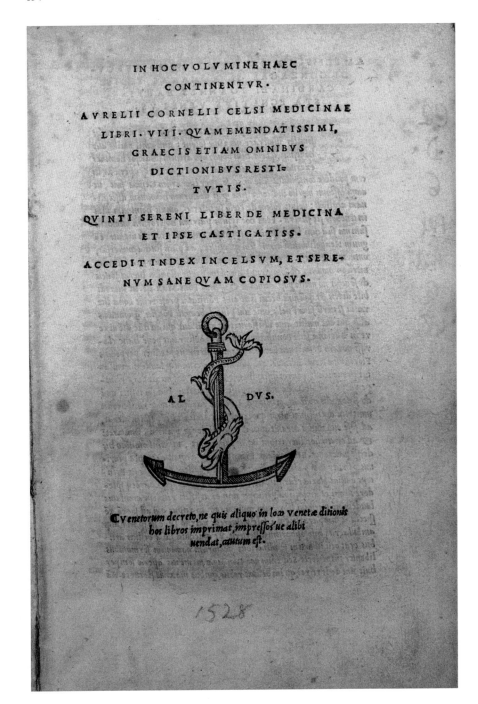

IN HOC VOLVMINE HAEC
CONTINENTVR.

AVRELII CORNELII CELSI MEDICINAE
LIBRI. VIII. QVAM EMENDATISSIMI,
GRAECIS ETIAM OMNIBVS
DICTIONIBVS RESTI=
TVTIS.

QVINTI SERENI LIBER DE MEDICINA
ET IPSE CASTIGATISS.

ACCEDIT INDEX IN CELSVM, ET SERE-
NVM SANE QVAM COPIOSVS.

AL   DVS.

Venetorum decreto, ne quis aliquo in loco venetæ ditionis
hos libros imprimat, impreſſos'ue alibi
uendat, cautum eſt.

1528

Fig. 8.2 De Medicina, book 8, by Aulus Cornelius Celsus [9]

What Are the Stories Behind Some Physicians and Scientists Who Became Very Involved in the Diseases They Studied?

Albert Hoffman, the man who synthesized lysergic acid diethylamide (LSD) in 1943, took the drug himself and recorded his strange visions. American scientist Jonas Salk tested his injectable polio vaccine on his wife, his children, and himself. Men and women who devote years of their lives to studying (and writing about) a particular disease, organism, or other phenomenon often become quite involved in the quest. Sometimes the search for answers prompts them to follow paths most of us would sensibly avoid, such as experiments on family members, co-workers, and themselves. Here are some of these tales—and misadventures. We know about them because the researchers (or those close to them) left us written records of what they did.

John Hunter (1728–1793)

Scottish surgeon and anatomist, sometimes called the father of scientific surgery, once told his student and friend Edward Jenner, "Don't think, try the experiment" [13] (see Fig. 8.3). John Hunter believed that gonorrhea and syphilis were a single affliction, and that a person could only suffer from one significant disease at a time [15]. Herein lies a tale that may or may not be true; there are vocal advocates for both versions. Wherever truth lies, it is a colorful story: In 1767, Hunter is reported to have performed an experiment in which he inoculated himself with gonorrhea.

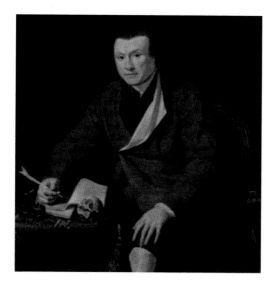

Fig. 8.3 Portrait of John Hunter by his brother-in-law, Robert Home, painted probably in 1784 [14]

Unfortunately the needle also contained the Spirochete of syphilis. When he contracted both diseases he concluded that, indeed, there was but one, single venereal disease [16]. In fact, the odds are that Hunter actually performed the experiment, but on someone other than himself.

In 1793 Hunter died in the boardroom of St. George Hospital. The next morning the anatomy students were more than mildly surprised to find the body on the dissecting table to be that of their teacher, Dr. Hunter. This was Hunter's final wish—to help his students learn anatomy [17].

Here is another colorful aside about Dr. Hunter. As an anatomist, he employed grave robbers, euphemistically called resurrectionists, to procure cadavers for dissection, and these dead bodies were delivered through the back door of the house. Hunter's home was the inspiration for the home of Dr. Jekyll in Robert Lewis Stevenson's 1886 novel *The Strange Case of Dr. Jekyll and Mr. Hyde*.

Paolo Mantegazza (1831–1910)

Italian neurologist Paolo Mantegazza returned from South America believing in the almost mystical properties of some ingestants, notably the stimulant powers of cocaine. He self-experimented by chewing coca leaves daily and then wrote a paper describing his conclusions [18]:

> "… I sneered at the poor mortals condemned to live in this valley of tears while I, carried on the wings of two leaves of coca, went flying through the spaces of 77,438 words, each more splendid than the one before…An hour later, I was sufficiently calm to write these words in a steady hand: God is unjust because he made man incapable of sustaining the effect of coca all life long. I would rather have a life span of ten years with coca than one of 10 000 000 000 000 000 000 000 centuries without coca."

William Beaumont (1785–1853)

In 1833, William Beaumont published the findings of a longitudinal study of the actions of gastric secretions and the physiology of digestion [19] (see Fig. 8.4). His observations were based on a series of one patient, but what a patient this was! While working in 1822 for the American Fur Company on Mackinac Island, a small island (about four square miles) in Lake Huron in Michigan, Alexis St. Martin sustained a shotgun blast to his anterior abdomen. Beaumont, a US Army surgeon and the physician on site, rendered treatment and, against all odds, St. Martin survived. The patient, however, was left with a persistent fistula into the stomach. This rendered St. Martin unfit for work, but an ideal subject to study the functioning of the stomach. Beaumont rescued his patient from unemployment by hiring him as a handyman, allowing the physician to continue experiments, such as inserting food with a string attached through the fistula, and then retrieving the food later to

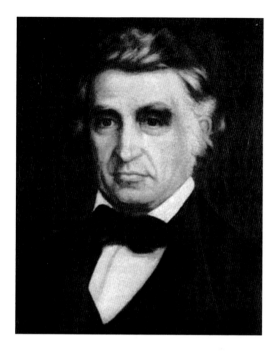

Fig. 8.4 William Beaumont, US Army surgeon who studied physiology of the stomach [20]

observe the state of digestion. These experiments continued off and on for 12 years, until Beaumont and St. Martin finally parted ways in 1834.

In the end, while making a house call, Beaumont slipped on icy steps and died in 1853. The more interesting backstories concern St. Martin, who outlived Beaumont by 27 years. In 1856, an entrepreneur describing himself as a doctor paraded St. Martin on a ten-city tour—not unlike the freak shows common in carnivals of the day. Following his death in 1880, the family of St. Martin left his body unburied until it decomposed in the sun and then buried the remains with rocks on the casket—all to discourage the "resurrectionists" [21].

Sir Patrick Manson (1844–1922)

Among those who studied malaria around the end of the nineteenth and beginning of the twentieth century was British physician Sir Patrick Manson. Thanks to his work on malaria and filariasis, Manson has been called "the father of tropical medicine" [22]. In the spirit of family experimentation of the time, Manson allowed malarious mosquitoes to bite his own son and another volunteer. Not surprisingly, both developed malaria. Manson then—successfully—treated both with quinine, and then went on to report his experiment in the *British Medical Journal* (BMJ) in 1900 [23].

Joseph Goldberger (1874–1929)

In the early twentieth century pellagra was rampant in the southern USA, and widely believed to be caused by a "germ," similar to tuberculosis, gonorrhea, and other communicable diseases of the day. In response to this public health hazard, in 1914 the US Surgeon General dispatched a United States Public Health (USPHS) physician named Joseph Goldberger to find the cause of pellagra and stamp it out (see Fig. 8.5).

Goldberger, however, postulated a theory that differed with the contemporary belief that a "germ" was the cause of pellagra after observing that, in mental hospitals and prisons, inmates often had pellagra and the staff did not. These two groups spent their days in close quarters, but one thing differed: their diets. In short, the inmates ate a diet consisting largely of corn products, while the staff ate a balanced diet that included fruits and vegetables. Goldberger postulated that pellagra was a dietary deficiency, and not due to a "germ" at all.

To prove his point—that there is no pellagra germ—Goldberger, his wife, and his assistant held "filth parties." They swabbed their own noses with material from the noses of pellagra patients, they swallowed pellagra scabs, and they injected themselves with blood from pellagra patients—the latter a practice I consider

Fig. 8.5 Joseph
Goldberger, US Public
Health Service physician
and epidemiologist [24]

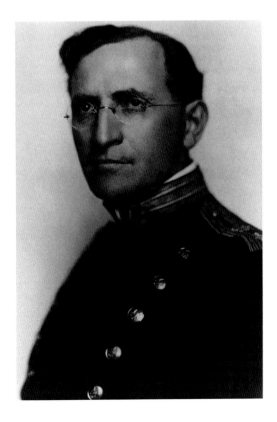

especially ill advised. No one developed pellagra, which today we know is actually a deficiency of niacin in the diet.

In 1922 Goldberger reported his findings in the *Journal of the American Medical Association* (JAMA) [25].

Barry Marshall (1951–)

In the early 1980s, Australian physicians Barry Marshall and Robin Warren postulated that peptic ulcer disease has a bacterial cause, specifically *H. pylori*, rather than being the result of excess gastric secretion, spicy food, and stress. Their theory about the relationship between *H. pylori* and peptic ulcer prompted skepticism among fellow physicians until Marshall took a bold step. He swallowed *H. pylori* organisms that had been cultured on a Petri dish. Within a few days he developed acute gastritis that yielded *H. pylori* on culture. Marshall's symptoms were subsequently treated successfully with antibiotics. In 1985, Marshall published the results of his self-experimentation [26]. He and Warren continued their experiments and reports, and, in 1951, were jointly awarded the Nobel Prize in Physiology or Medicine.

Here is an update on Marshall's research (see Fig. 8.6). He is now working on a way to use *H. pylori* as a vehicle to carry the human immunodeficiency virus (HIV) into the stomach, where it may stay long enough to generate antibodies and serve as a vaccine against acquired immunodeficiency disease (AIDS) [28].

What May Be the Most Cited of All Medical Articles and What Is the Story Behind the Author?

According to one source [29], Francis Weld Peabody's *The Care of the Patient* is the most cited article in the medical literature, although such primacy is open to dispute. Yet, that this article is singled out among all the groundbreaking reports that have

Fig. 8.6 Australian gastroenterologist and Nobel laureate Barry Marshall. Photo credit: Barjammar [27]

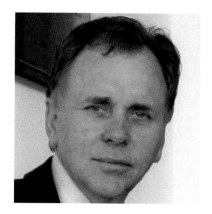

been published is remarkable when one considers that Peabody's essay deals exclusively with the interpersonal aspects of medicine and not with disease diagnosis or therapy [30].

This article, which ends with the often-quoted line, "the secret of the care of the patient is in caring for the patient," evolved from a series of lectures Peabody gave to the Harvard Medical School students in 1926. While giving these lectures, Peabody was aware that he had incurable sarcoma. A writer until the end, while taking analgesics at the end of life in 1927, Peabody penned an (unpublished) essay titled "Notes on the Effects of Morphine" [31].

Who Are Some Medical Writers Who Famously Faced Rejection?

In Chap. 5 I told of how, before its publication in 1796, Jenner's paper *An Inquiry into the Causes and Effects of the Variolae Vaccinae* was initially rejected by the Royal Society, and how in 1847 the world was not ready to embrace Ignaz Semmelweis' writings on hand washing. Through the years, there is a proud history of rejection of early submissions of works by medical writers. Here are three examples:

Frank Gill Slaughter (1908–2001)

Frank G. Slaughter was a graduate of Johns Hopkins University Medical School and a board-certified surgeon, but success as a writer did not come easily. While working as a surgeon, he began writing on a $60 typewriter he was paying off at a rate of $5 per month. At first he wrote a number of short stories, but sold only one. One of Slaughter's patients at the time, a Pulitzer Prize-winning author, read his work and advised him, "Stick to operating." I wonder: Was this testimony praise of Slaughter's surgical skill or a commentary on his writing?

But Slaughter soldiered on, writing the semiautobiographical first novel *That None Should Die*, published by Doubleday in 1941 after five earlier rejections. Frank G. Slaughter eventually turned from surgery to writing following the initial success of his first novel and the four books that followed. Eventually his books would sell more than 60 million copies [32].

Howard F. Conn (1908–1982)

No one wanted to listen to Dr. Conn in 1946. After all, Howard F. Conn was not a professor of medicine; he wasn't even on a medical school faculty. In fact, he had never even served a residency in a medical specialty. He did not have a curriculum vita listing numerous prestigious publications. He had never written or edited a book. He was just a small-town general practitioner from Uniontown, PA, who had recently been discharged from the army. He was an unlikely candidate for a role as reference book editor. But Dr. Conn had an idea.

He contacted several medical publishers, but to no avail. Finally he found his way to Saunders Publishers in Philadelphia. Here, according to a story related to me about three decades ago by my own Saunders editor, Al Meier, Conn got lucky. It seems that there was a new, young Saunders editor, one that wasn't busy yet. Someone said, "Let the new editor talk to this Dr. Conn." The new editor listened, and understood the potential of a large reference book, produced yearly, that contained the therapeutic recommendations of a host of invited specialists, and that covered most diseases commonly seen by generalists. At this meeting, *Current Therapy* was born.

When Conn died in 1982, the book, in annual editions, had sold more than one million copies. *Conn's Current Therapy* continues today, now with its third and fourth editors, retaining the same model proposed originally to a prescient young editor in Philadelphia [33].

As a bonus, here is backstory about Doctor Howard Conn. He served as a Battalion Surgeon in the US Army in Europe during World War II, and was the model for the empathic and trusted army doctor in the 1945 book *Up Front* by "Willie and Joe" cartoonist Bill Maudlin [33].

H. Richard Hornberger (1924–1997)

Following his service at the 8055th Mobile Army Surgical Hospital in Korea, H. Richard Hornberger of Crabapple Cove in Bremen, Maine, opened his thoracic surgery practice and, in his spare time, wrote a novel about his experiences in the service. As is usual with first-time authors and first novels, the manuscript suffered many rejections. Eventually, sportswriter W.C. Heinz helped Hornberger revise the novel. After 8 years of seeking a publisher, Hornberger finally saw his book published as *MASH: A Novel About Three Army Doctors*, with Hornberger listed as author under the pseudonym Richard Hooker.

After the book came the movie starring Alan Alda as Hawkeye Pierce. The movie rights were sold for a pittance and, according to Baxter, Hornberger was "so furious at having sold the film rights for only a few hundred dollars that he never again signed a copy of the book" [34]. But we should not shed tears for Hornberger/Hooker. The film was followed by a long-running television series, bringing the angry author a sizeable royalty payment every time you or I viewed an episode.

The Richard Hooker pen name anecdote is this: The author chose his pseudonym to describe his golf game [35].

What Medical Writers Suffered Health Problems That May Have Influenced Their Lives and Their Writing?

Many writers of all genres have had physical illness that influenced their writing. Lewis Carroll, in fact the pen name of English cleric and author Charles Lutwidge Dodgson (1832–1898), suffered from migraine headache with aura characterized by fortification spectra; these visual manifestations may have been the basis of the distorted figures in his "Alice" books [36]. Scottish author Robert Lewis Stevenson (1850–1894) suffered from persistent chronic lung disease, probably tuberculosis or bronchiectasis. His gratitude to his physicians prompted him to write his famous ode to physicians, *The Doctor*, that begins: "There are men and classes of men that stand above the common herd; the soldier, the sailor, and the shepherd not infrequently; the artist rarely; rarer still the clergyman; the physician almost as a rule …" [37]. The following are some medical writers whose work—clinical care, research, or writing—may have been affected by their diseases.

William Carlos Williams (1883–1963)

William Carlos Williams, the physician-poet of Rutherford, NJ, the doctor who saw patients by day and wrote poetry at night, suffered a heart attack in 1948 followed by a debilitating series of strokes beginning the next year. This limited his "doctoring," and he retired from medicine in 1951. Yet he spoke enthusiastically about his newfound free time to read and the "opportunity for thought." Following his strokes Williams did some of his best writing until his death in 1963 [38, 39].

Archie Cochrane (1909–1988)

Archie Cochrane, for whom the Cochrane Coalition is named, was a British epidemiologist who championed the randomized controlled trial in medicine. He was the author of a 1971 monograph *Effectiveness and Efficiency*, in which he denounced the quality of British health care of his time. Cochrane suffered from porphyria, the same disease that afflicted King George III—"Mad King George"—in the eighteenth century. According to Shah et al., Cochrane's porphyria "played a significant role in his professional views," which just might refer to his criticism of the medical care rendered by his contemporaries [40].

Alex Comfort (1920–2000)

While at Highgate School in London, British physician, scientist, and author Alex Comfort destroyed most of his left hand in an ill-advised chemistry experiment involving the ingredients in gunpowder. Only his left thumb remained. Comfort, however, adopted a positive attitude toward his disability, reportedly using the deformed digit to advantage when performing uterine inversions.

We remember Comfort, not for his prowess in the operating theater or delivery room, but for his 1972 best-selling book *The Joy of Sex*. In 1997, an abbreviated edition titled *The Joy of Sex, the Pocket Edition* was honored with the Bookseller Magazine Prize for Oddest Title of the Year [41].

Edward Rosenbaum (1915–2009)

Found to have cancer of the larynx at age 70, Dr. Rosenbaum wrote a book—*A Taste of My Own Medicine: When the Doctor Is the Patient*—telling what can happen when a doctor suffers from a serious illness. He describes an Odyssey of tests, decisions, delays, indifference, and humiliation. Dr. Rosenbaum died in 2009, but his message lives on in his book. The book was followed by a 1991 movie, titled *The Doctor*, starring William Hurt as Rosenbaum [42].

Oliver Sacks (1933–)

British-American neurologist Oliver Sacks, winner of the 2001 Lewis Thomas Prize for Writing about Science, often writes of individuals who suffer from uncommon neurologic diseases. Sacks, himself, suffers from prosopagnosia, aka face blindness, the inability to recognize the faces of familiar persons [43].

The title chapter of his book *The Man Who Mistook His Wife for a Hat* describes someone with visual agnosia, similar to the ailment Sacks suffers [44]. His book *The Island of the Colorblind* tells of an island where most of the inhabitants have achromatopsia, a type of reduced visual acuity, difficulty seeing in bright light, and inability to discern colors. Also, Sacks' first published book (1970) was titled *Migraine: Evolution of a Common Disorder*, presumably describing another of the author's ailments.

Adeline Yen Mah (1937–)

Chinese-American physician and author Adeline Yen Mah grew up in the Republic of China. Her mother died as a complication of her birth, and hence the child was considered "bad luck" by the family. Yen Mah was raised chiefly by her stepmother, at whose hands she suffered physical and emotional abuse. The author describes these experiences in her autobiographical books *Falling Leaves* (1997) and *Chinese Cinderella* (1999), both of which have sold more than a million copies [45].

David Hilfiker (1947–)

Despite a warning about risking "serious damage to his career," family physician David Hilfiker wrote a 1984 article titled "Facing our Mistakes," reporting some of his own clinical errors, which was published in the NEJM [46]. This was followed by his book *Healing the Wounds: A Physician Looks at His Work*, which brought Hilfiker national attention as a serious medical writer [47].

Hilfiker's personal medical adventures and his ongoing progress notes, recorded in his blog, are a roller-coaster saga. He was diagnosed in September 2012 with cognitive impairment, probably Alzheimer disease, a journey he chronicled on his blog as "watching the lights go out." A year later the Alzheimer label was changed to "subjective cognitive complaints." As I write this chapter, Hilfiker's symptoms seem to have stabilized: "My cognitive lights are no longer winking out." He is closing his blog after bringing insights about cognitive impairment to many readers [48].

Charles Krauthammer (1950–)

Many don't know that Charles Krauthammer, Pulitzer Prize-winning columnist and political commentator often seen on television, is also a physician. His personal health story is that, during his first year at Harvard Medical School, Krauthammer suffered a diving-board accident and, since then, has been paralyzed and confined to a wheelchair. He somehow finished his medical school studies, graduated, and served a psychiatric residency at Massachusetts General Hospital. While still a resident in 1978, he was lead author on a paper describing the concept of "secondary mania," occurring due to drugs, infection, neoplasm, epilepsy, and metabolic disturbances. In their paper, the authors postulate: "Furthermore, the concept of secondary mania casts doubt on any unitary or single-agent hypothesis of the etiology of mania and supports the notion of a continuum of psychopathologic syndromes" [49].

Eben Alexander III (1953–)

In 2008, American neurosurgeon Eben Alexander III acquired a rare disease: *E. coli* meningitis. The infection resulted in a prolonged coma, during which Alexander reports heavenly perceptions, which he describes as "seeing the other side." His book, *Proof of Heaven: A Neurosurgeon's Journey into the Afterlife,* tells of his out-of-body and near-death experience [50]. The book was on the *New York Times* best-seller list for 97 weeks.

Alexander's literary success has been tarnished by reports of malpractice cases, alterations in a surgical report, and termination of hospital privileges [51]. The book, nevertheless, is a huge success, and Dr. Alexander has become a physician-writer celebrity.

Who Were Some Medical Writers Whose Family Members or Spouses Were Influential, Sometimes Partners, in Their Writing?

Writing is often a family event, and countless spouses have conducted research, provided critical readings, offered suggestions for manuscript improvement, reviewed page proofs, and offered consolation when unfavorable reviews were published. Most of these loyal spouses and family members were thanked in the Acknowledgement sections; some even had their name on book covers as coauthors. Here are a few of each:

- **Marie and Pierre Curie**: Together Marie and Pierre discovered radium and published papers describing the element polonium (named for Marie's home country, Poland) and radium (from the word "ray"); they coined the word "radioactivity" (see Fig. 8.7). The Curies were both frugal and committed. The dark blue lab dress Marie wore for years had originally been her wedding dress, and the Curies used all their Nobel Prize money to support their ongoing research. The partnership ended in 1906 when Pierre was killed after being struck by a horse-drawn vehicle. Five years later, Marie Curie became the first person to ever be awarded a second Nobel Prize [53].
- **William H. Masters and Virginia E. Johnson**: The Masters and Johnson research team brought the topic of sex to the American reading audience with their 1966 book *Human Sexual Response* [54]. Virginia, first hired in 1957 as Johnson's research assistant, married him in 1971; thus technically, she was neither spouse nor kin when *Human Sexual Response* was first published. The Masters and Johnson marriage ended in divorce in 1992.

Fig. 8.7 Marie and Pierre Curie in their laboratory. Source: Vitold Muratov, author. Welt im Umbruch 1900–1914. Stuttgart: Verlag Das Beste. GmbH. 1999 [52]

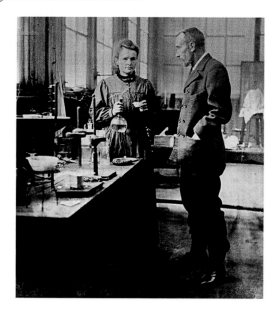

- **Janet Jeppson and Isaac Asimov**: In 1970, American psychiatrist Janet Opal Jeppson began writing children's science fiction books. Then, following her marriage to Isaac Asimov in 1973 they became true writing partners, and coauthored several books together, including one of my favorites, *How To Enjoy Writing: A Book of Aid and Comfort*, published in 1987 [55].
- **David and Vera Mace**: David and Vera Mace wrote *How to Have a Happy Marriage*, published in 1977. Dr. David Mace was professor of family sociology at Wake Forest University School of Medicine. The Maces founded the Association for Couples in Marriage Enrichment and wrote more than 30 books on marriage and the family.
- **Pamela Hartzband and Jerome Groopman**: Both physicians and married to one another, Groopman and Hartzband collaborated on the 2011 book, *Your Medical Mind: How to Decide What Is Right for You*, a sequel to Groopman's 2007 bestseller *How Doctors Think* [56].
- **Howard W. Jones and Georgeanna Seegar Jones**: This husband and wife team, both specialists in reproductive gynecology, were subject to age-related mandatory retirement at Johns Hopkins School of Medicine. They moved to Norfolk, Virginia, and joined the faculty of Eastern Virginia Medical School (EVMS), the medical school where my wife and I hold faculty appointments. Here the Joneses began the in vitro fertilization (IVF) program that led to the birth of the America's first "test tube baby" in 1981. (The world's first IVF baby was born in England in 1978.) Although Georgeanna died of Alzheimer disease in 2005, Howard continues his academic career and in 2015, at age 104, he published his 12th book, titled *In Vitro Fertilization Comes to America* [57].

Who Are Some Medical Writers Who Penned Books on Religious Topics?

Some writers, such as Eben Alexander III, mentioned above, write on spiritual themes, sometimes with a "medical" slant, sometimes not.

- **Sir Thomas Browne**: In the seventeenth century, English physician writer Sir Thomas Browne wrote *Religio Medici (The Religion of a Physician)*, published in 1643 (see Fig. 8.8). The work described some notions that were in conflict with religious dogma of the day, causing controversy that led the book to become a best seller [59].
- **Albert Schweitzer**: Physician, philosopher, and theologian Albert Schweitzer (see Fig. 8.9). We know him because of his service in what is now Gabon, in Africa. But before his years as a medical missionary, Schweitzer's reputation had been previously established with the publication of his book *Geschichte der Leben-Jesu-Forschung* ("history of life-of-Jesus research") in 1906, subsequently translated into English, and published as *The Quest of the Historical Jesus* [61].

Fig. 8.8 English physician and author Thomas Browne. Photo source: Popular Science Monthly Volume 50 [58]

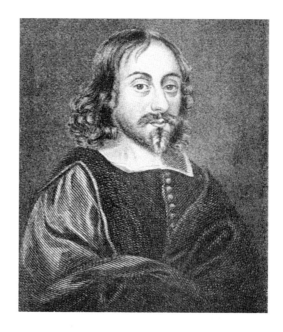

Fig. 8.9 Nobel laureate Albert Schweitzer, 1965. Source Dutch National Archives [60]

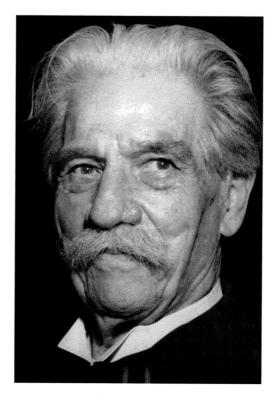

- **Francis Collins**: Physician-geneticist Francis Collins, currently Director of the National Institutes of Health in Bethesda, Maryland, led the group that brought the Human Genome Project to a successful completion. His 2006 best-selling book, titled *The Language of God: A Scientist Presents Evidence for Belief*, describes his belief in a theistic evolution [62].

Do Medical Writers Ever Use Pseudonyms?

I mentioned earlier that Richard Hooker was the pen name assumed by H. Richard Hornberger, author of *MASH: A Novel About Three Army Doctors*. And while you may or may not consider Benjamin Franklin a medical author, he did write *Some Account of the Success of Inoculation for the Small-Pox in England and America*, and he invented the urethral catheter and bifocal glasses. Franklin wrote under a host of pseudonyms: Silence Dogood, Alice Addertongue, Celia Single, Anthony Afterwit, Pennsylvanus, Philomath, Homespun, A Traveler, Pacificus Secundus, and, of course, Poor Richard, the latter apparently an echo of the name Richard Saunders, a late seventeenth-century English almanac writer [63]. Can you identify the true identity of the following pseudonyms used by medical writers. The answers are given below:

A. Alcofribas Nasier
B. A.C. Smith
C. Samuel Shem
D. Old Hubert
E. John Lange
F. Egerton Yorrick Davis

Here are the true identities, physicians all:

A. Alcofribas Nasier is the pen name used by François Rabelais, sixteenth-century author of *Gargantua and Pantagruel*. The pen name is an anagram of the author's true name, François Rabelais (lacking only the cedilla on the "c"). Rabelais published his first two books, which were likely to be condemned by the church, under the pseudonym. His third book was published under his own name [64].
B. A.C. Smith was a name used by Sir Arthur Conan Doyle, the creator of Sherlock Holmes, when he played for the Portsmouth Association Football Club.
C. When I first read *The House of God* in 1978, I knew that Samuel Shem was a pseudonym. We later learned that the book had been written by American psychiatrist Stephen Joseph Bergman.
D. In the nineteenth century, James Parkinson wrote *On Chorea*, describing the disease later named Parkinson disease in his memory. In the period following the French Revolution, he wrote a number of controversial pamphlets under the name "Old Hubert" [65].

E. The early works of Michael Crichton, author of *Jurassic Park* and *The Andromeda Strain,* appeared under the pseudonym, John Lange. *Lang* means long in German. Crichton was very tall: 6 ft, 9 in.

F. Egerton Yorrick Davis was the alter ego of none other than teacher, aphorist, and medical writer Sir William Osler, who sometimes signed into conferences and hotels using this name. "Davis" authored several waggish letters and reports, one describing "an uncommon form of vaginismus" causing "*penis captivus*" that required treatment with chloroform [66].

What Are Some Other Lesser Known Facts About Famous Medical Writers and Writing?

Erasmus Darwin (1731–1802)

Erasmus Darwin, an English practicing physician and writer, was the father of Robert Darwin, also a physician, and the grandfather of Charles Darwin, author of *On the Origin of Species* in 1859. Erasmus Darwin was the author of *Zoonomia: The Laws of Organic Life*, *The Botanic Garden*, and *The Temple of Nature*. In his spare time he invented a copying machine, a canal lift for barges, a weather-monitoring machine, and a steering mechanism for his carriage that predated what would be used in automobiles more than a century later. Grandson Charles Darwin was supposed to become a physician but changed his profession direction because he could not bear the cries of the suffering [67].

Jean-Paul Marat (1743–1793)

Physician Jean-Paul Marat is remembered for his outspoken writings during the French Revolution that began in 1789 and lasted for a decade. Marat championed the *Sans-Culottes*—a radical partisan group that took their name from their rejection of the culottes (knee breeches) affected by foppish gentlemen of the time [68].

Les Sans Culottes was one of my favorite restaurants in New York City, right in the theater district. I am sad to report that it closed in 2014.

Mungo Park (1771–1806)

Scottish physician and explorer Mungo Park, author of a book titled *Travels in the Interior Districts of Africa* (1799), is believed to be the first European to explore the central region of the River Niger in Western Africa. One of the earliest and best of the travel writers, Park told his readers of the wonders found in a large and mostly unexplored continent [69].

David Livingstone (1813–1873)

Scottish medical missionary David Livingstone, famously made a journey across Africa from the Atlantic to the Indian Ocean in 1854–1856, and then seemed to disappear into the wilds of the so-called dark continent. Eventually the New York Herald newspaper dispatched Henry Morton Stanley to find him. At their famous meeting on November 10, 1871, Stanley reportedly asked, "Dr. Livingstone, I presume." The question, if asked at all, would have seemed somewhat superfluous, since Stanley had just encountered the only non-African within hundreds of miles. Livingstone's most important writing was his *Field Diary*, which is available online [70]. He has been eponymously honored in the name of the Livingstone fruit bat, *Pteropus livingstonii*.

Sir Ronald Ross (1857–1932)

Indian-born British physician Sir Ronald Ross was, like William Carlos Williams, who would come later, both a doctor and a poet. Ross would memorialize important life events with poems (see Fig. 8.10). Some of these are found in his book *Selected Poems*, published in 1928. In 1897 he showed mosquitoes to be the vector of malaria

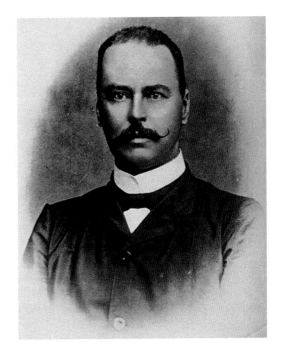

Fig. 8.10 Sir Ronald Ross, whose discovery of the malaria parasite in the gastrointestinal tract of a mosquito demonstrated the way that malaria is transmitted. This file comes from Wellcome Images, a website operated by Wellcome Trust, a global charitable foundation based in the UK [71]

by finding the parasite in the insect's gastrointestinal tract [72]. Shortly following the discovery he began to compose a poem to commemorate the event:

This day relenting God
Hath placed within my hand
A wondrous thing; and God
Be praised. At His command,
Seeking His secret deeds
With tears and toiling breath,
I find thy cunning seeds,
O million-murdering Death.
I know this little thing
A myriad men will save.
O Death, where is thy sting?
Thy victory, O Grave?

Ross's work helping us to understand the life cycle of the malarial parasite set the stage for mosquito control efforts that have saved countless lives, helped build the Panama Canal beginning in 1904, and earned him the 1902 Nobel Prize for Physiology or Medicine.

Osamu Tezuka (1928–1989)

This Japanese physician holds a distinction perhaps no other medical writer can duplicate: He had a successful career as a cartoonist. The creator of comic series Kimba the White Lion, Black Jack, and Astro Boy, Tezuka is seen as the "Japanese Walt Disney" [73].

Silas Weir Mitchell (1829–1914)

An American physician and writer, remembered for his description of causalgia and considered by some to be the "father of neurology," was a champion of the "rest cure," which he considered especially useful for patients with neurasthenia [74]. His remedy included confinement to bed in solitude. An acknowledged expert in his field, Mitchell was consulted by Virginia Woolf, who later wrote of his rest cure, "you invoke proportion; order rest in bed; rest in solitude; silence and rest; rest without friends, without books, without messages; 6 months rest; until a man who went in weighing seven stone six comes out weighing twelve" [75].

Havelock Ellis (1859–1940)

British physician-author Havelock Ellis, together with John Addington Symonds, wrote the first objective monograph on homosexuality, titled *Sexual Inversion*, and published in English in 1897 [76]. The book was groundbreaking in that it did not describe homosexuality as a perversion or a crime. Ellis decried the use of the word "homosexual," stating, "'Homosexual' is a barbarously hybrid word, and I claim no responsibility for it. It is, however, convenient, and now widely used. 'Homogenic' has been suggested as a substitute" [77].

But Ellis did not stop there. He went on to write *Sexual Selection in Man* (1905), *Sex in Relation to Society* (1910), and *The Problem of Race-Regeneration* (1911). Ellis, however, was a strong supporter of eugenics, and the work that remains most controversial is his commentary on what he terms social hygiene, meaning maintaining the optimization of the race. In this book, titled *The Task of Social Hygiene* [78], he writes:

> Eventually, it seems evident, a general system, whether private or public, whereby all personal facts, biological and mental, normal and morbid, are duly and systematically registered, must become inevitable if we are to have a real guide as to those persons who are most fit, or most unfit to carry on the race.

Later, when the Nazi Party in Germany advocated sterilization of "undesirables," Ellis considered this position to be scientifically sound and did not raise his voice in protest [79].

W. Somerset Maugham (1874–1965)

Recalled as a prolific writer, and an almost incidentally as a physician, W. Somerset Maugham authored such memorable works as *Of Human Bondage* (1915), *The Moon and Sixpence* (1919), *The Painted Veil* (1925), and *The Razor's Edge* (1944). He also wrote short stories and plays such as *East of Suez* (1922) and *For Services Rendered* (1932).

During World War I, Maugham was sent to Russia on a spy mission by the British Secret Intelligence Service (which we now know as MI6). His task was to counter German pacifist propaganda regarding the war and do what he could to thwart the threatened Bolshevik takeover of the government, the latter proving to be a futile endeavor. Later the author put his experience to good use, however, building on what he had learned about espionage to write a tale of a decidedly urbane spy. The book was titled *Ashenden: Or the British Agent,* and the title character may have been the inspiration for Ian Fleming's Agent 007, aka James Bond [80].

A.J. Cronin (1896–1981)

If one were to seek the inspiration for the British National Health Service, established in 1948, the search would probably lead to A.J. Cronin and his book *The Citadel*, published in 1937 [81]. In this book, Cronin calls upon personal experiences as he chronicles the life of Andrew Manson, a young doctor serving a struggling Welsh mining village and who later moves on to become an affluent London practitioner. Cronin's story highlighted the disparities in health care received by the poor versus the wealthy in Britain, and the widely read novel helped bolster popular support for nationalization of the British health care system a decade later.

Lewis Thomas (1913–1993)

If Lewis Thomas were alive today would he prefer to be remembered as a clinical researcher, an administrator, or an author? After helping to finance his medical school education by selling blood and publishing poems in popular magazines such as *Saturday Evening Post* and *Harper's Bazaar*, he went on to a distinguished career, which included groundbreaking immunologic research. Thomas served as dean of both New York University and Yale schools of medicine and as president of Sloan-Kettering Research Institute. He authored scientific papers and also a series of essays published in the *New England Journal of Medicine*, the latter subsequently published as *The Lives of a Cell* (New York: Viking; 1974) and as *The Medusa and the Snail: More Notes of a Biology Watcher* (New York: Viking; 1979). Never one to take the common path, his death in 1993 was caused by Waldenstrom lymphoma, a rare type of B-cell lymphoma [82].

Elisabeth Kübler-Ross (1926–2004)

The name of American psychiatrist Elisabeth Kübler-Ross became widely known following the 1969 publication of her book *On Death and Dying*, in which she described the five stages of grief: denial, anger, bargaining, depression, and acceptance (see Fig. 8.11). Here are three things you probably did not know about Kübler-Ross [84]:

- **Birth**: She was born in Switzerland, the middle of triplet girls.
- **Career**: Despite her father's objections, she sought a career in medicine. Because of being pregnant at the time, she was denied a pediatric residency, and instead became a psychiatrist.
- **Late life**: Following the success of *On Death and Dying*, in her later years Kübler-Ross focused her attentions on the supernatural and the quest for communication with the dead.

Atul Gawande (1965–)

Just as A.J. Cronin's writing may have helped foster the establishment of the National Health in Britain, an article by American surgeon and *New Yorker* medical writer Atul Gawande influenced thinking about America's Affordable Care Act of 2010.

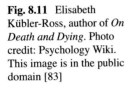

Fig. 8.11 Elisabeth Kübler-Ross, author of *On Death and Dying*. Photo credit: Psychology Wiki. This image is in the public domain [83]

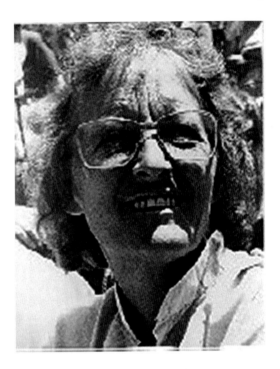

The article titled *The Cost Conundrum—What a Texas Town Can Teach Us About Health Care* compared the high cost of health care in a Texas town to the lower cost of care in a setting with increased emphasis on better care for less cost [85]. Pear tells us that President Obama read the article and cited it to colleagues as "what we've got to fix" [86].

In addition to his influence on national health policy, Gawande is known for his books, which include *Complications: A Surgeon's Notes on an Imperfect Science* (2002) and *The Checklist Manifesto: How to Get Things Right* (2009).

What Is the All-Time Best-Selling Book by a Medical Writer?

According to Maier, the laurels go to *The Common Sense Book of Baby and Child Care* by American pediatrician Benjamin Spock. Published in 1946, this guide for the parents of young children has sold more than 50 million copies [87] (see Fig. 8.12). It is not, however, close to being the best-selling book of all time and is eclipsed by such works as *A Tale of Two Cities* (Charles Dickens, 1859), *And Then There None* (Agatha Christie, 1939), and *Harry Potter and the Philosopher's Stone* (J.K. Rowling, 1997), all enjoying sales of more than a 100 million copies [89].

Fig. 8.12 Benjamin
Spock, American
pediatrician (with his first
granddaughter, Susannah).
Photo credit: Thomas
R. Koeniges, Look
magazine photo collection
[88]

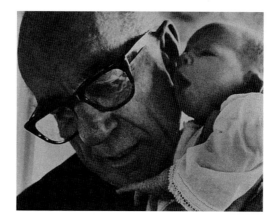

References

1. Flexner JT. Washington: the indispensable man. Boston: Little, Brown; 1974.
2. Lewiston Daily Sun, 11 Oct 1928. Available at: http://news.google.com/newspapers?nid=192 8&dat=19281011&id=vxggAAAAIBAJ&sjid=eWYFAAAAIBAJ&pg=4604,938276.
3. Thatcher M. The path to power. New York: Harper Collins; 1995.
4. Imhotep-Louvre.jpg. This file is licensed under the Creative Commons Attribution-Share Alike 3.0 Unported license. Available at: http://commons.wikimedia.org/wiki/File:Imhotep-Louvre.JPG.
5. Osler W. A series of lectures delivered at Yale University, Apr 1913. Available at: http://www. gutenberg.org/files/1566/1566-h/1566-h.htm.
6. Kemp BJ. Ancient Egypt. New York: Routledge; 2005.
7. Langslow DR. Medical Latin in the Roman Empire. New York: Oxford University Press; 2000.
8. Norman J. The oldest western medical document after the Hippocratic writings, and how it survived the middle ages. Available at: http://www.historyofinformation.com/expanded. php?id=2111.
9. De medicina V 00117 00000006.tif. This work is in the public domain in the United States and those countries with a copyright term of the life of the author plus 100 years or less. Available at: http://commons.wikimedia.org/wiki/File:De_medicina_V00117_00000006.tif.
10. Buckley K. The most important article in NEJM history. Now@NEJM. Available at: http:// blogs.nejm.org/now/index.php/the-most-important-article-in-nejm-history/2012/11/01/.
11. Bigelow HJ. Insensibility during surgical operations produced by inhalation. Boston Med Surg J. 1846;XXXV(16):309. doi:10.1056/NEJM184611180351601.
12. Smith S. The ether patent. Med Times. 1862;4:83.
13. Kelly K. Old world and new; early medical care, 1700–1840. New York: Infobase; 2010.
14. John Hunter by Robert Home (about 1770).png. This work is in the public domain in the United States and those countries with a copyright term of the life of the author plus 100 years or less. Available at: http://commons.wikimedia.org/wiki/File:John_Hunter_by_Robert_Home_(about_1770).png.
15. Hunter J. A treatise on the venereal disease. London: G Nicole and J Johnson; 1786.
16. Wright DJ. John Hunter and the venereal disease. Ann R Coll Surg Engl. 1981;63:198.
17. Moore W. John Hunter: 1728–93. James Lind Library Bulletin: commentaries on the history of treatment evaluation. Available at: http://www.jameslindlibrary.org/illustrating/articles/john-hunter-1728-93.

18. Mantegazza P. *Sulle Virtù Igieniche e Medicinali della Coca e sugli Alimenti Nervosi* (On the hygienic and medicinal properties of coca and on nervine nourishment in general). Ann Univ Med. 1859;167:449.
19. Beaumont W. Experiments and observations on the gastric juice and the physiology of digestion. Printed by F.P. Allen; 1838.
20. William Beaumont.jpg. This image is in the public domain because its copyright has expired. Available at: http://commons.wikimedia.org/wiki/File:William_Beaumont.jpg.
21. Edwards E. The gruesome medical breakthrough of Dr. William Beaumont on Mackinac Island. Available at: http://mynorth.com/2010/05/the-gruesome-medical-breakthrough-of-dr-william-beaumont-on-mackinac-island/.
22. Chernin E. Patrick Manson and the transmission of filariasis. Am J Trop Med Hyg. 1977;25:1065.
23. Manson P. Experimental proof of the mosquito-malaria theory. BMJ. 1900;2:949. Available at: http://www.jameslindlibrary.org/illustrating/articles/john-hunter-1728-93.
24. Joseph Goldberger 01.jpg. This image is a work of the Centers for Disease Control and Prevention, part of the United States Department of Health and Human Services, taken or made as part of an employee's official duties. As a work of the U.S. federal government, the image is in the public domain. Available at: http://commons.wikimedia.org/wiki/File:Joseph_Goldberger_01.jpg.
25. Goldberger J. The relation of diet to pellagra. JAMA. 1922;78:1676. Available at: http://jama.jamanetwork.com/article.aspx?articleid=229937.
26. Marshall BJ. The pathogenesis of non-ulcer dyspepsia. Med J Aust. 1985;143:319.
27. Marshall 2008.jpg. The author has released this work into the public domain. Available at: http://commons.wikimedia.org/wiki/File:Marshall_2008.JPG.
28. Marshall B. Edible vaccines could help eradicate disease in the developing world. The Conversation. Available at: http://theconversation.com/edible-vaccines-could-help-eradicate-disease-in-the-developing-world-2204.
29. The care of the patient by F.W. Peabody. Cell2Soul: The Humane Health Care Blog. Available at: http://cell2soul.typepad.com/cell2soul_blog/2009/04/the-care-of-the-patient-by-fw-peabody.html.
30. Peabody FW. The care of the patient. JAMA. 1927;88:877. Available at: http://cell2soul.typepad.com/files/the_care_of_the_patient-1.pdf.
31. Peabody FW. Notes on the effect of morphine. Unpublished. Available at: http://cell2soul.typepad.com/cell2soul_blog/files/peabody_on_morphine.pdf.
32. Frank G(ill) Slaughter, pseudonym C.V. Terry. Available at: http://www.kirjasto.sci.fi/slaugh.htm.
33. Bope ET, Kellerman RD. Preface. Bope and Kellerman Conn's current therapy 2014. Available at: http://www.mdconsult.com/books/page.do?eid=4-u1.0-B978-1-4557-0296-1..09988-7&isbn=978-1-4557-0296-1&type=bookPage&from=content&uniqId=471542969-2.
34. Baxter J. A pound of paper: confessions of a book addict. New York: St. Martin's; 2005.
35. The story behind MASH. Available at: http://www.amarketingexpert.com/the-story-behind-mash/#sthash.hcQHMAyJ.dpuf.
36. Podoll K et al. Lewis Carroll's migraine experiences. Lancet. 1999;353:9161.
37. Stevenson RL. Dedication: underwoods. New York: Peter Fenelon Collier; 1887.
38. William Carlos Williams. The Poetry Foundation. Available at: http://www.poetryfoundation.org/bio/william-carlos-williams.
39. Williams WC. Paterson. New York: New Directions; 1963.
40. Shah HM et al. Archie Cochrane and his vision for evidence-based medicine. Plast Reconstr Surg. 2009;124:982.
41. The oddest book titles. Available at: http://people.sc.fsu.edu/~jburkardt/fun/wordplay/title_oddest.html.
42. Rosenbaum E. A taste of my own medicine: when the doctor is the patient. New York: Random House; 1988.

43. Katz N. Prosopagnosia: Oliver Sacks' battle with "face blindness." CBSnews.com; 26 Aug 2010. Available at: http://www.cbsnews.com/news/prosopagnosia-oliver-sacks-battle-with-face-blindness/.

44. Sacks O. The man who mistook his wife for a hat. New York: Touchstone; 1985.

45. Adeline Yen Mah. BBC. Available at: http://www.bbc.co.uk/worldservice/learningenglish/movingwords/celebritychoice/adelineyenmah.shtml.

46. Hilfiker D. Facing our mistakes. N Engl J Med. 1984;310:118.

47. Hilfiker D. Healing the wounds: a physician looks at his work. New York: Pantheon; 1985.

48. Hilfiker D. Watching the lights go out. Available at: http://davidhilfiker.blogspot.com/.

49. Krauthammer C et al. Secondary mania manic syndromes associated with antecedent physical illness or drugs. Arch Gen Psychiatry. 1978;35:1333.

50. Alexander E. Proof of Heaven: a neurosurgeon's journey into the afterlife. New York: Simon and Schuster; 2012.

51. Dittrich L. The prophet: an investigation into Eben Alexander, author of the blockbuster "Proof of Heaven". Esquire Magazine, Aug 2013; pp. 88–95.

52. Marie et Pierre Curie.jpg. This file is licensed under the Creative Commons Attribution-Share Alike 3.0 Unported license. Available at: http://commons.wikimedia.org/wiki/File:Marie_et_Pierre_Curie.jpg.

53. Goldsmith B. Obsessive genius: the inner world of Marie Curie. New York: Norton; 2005.

54. Masters WH, Johnson VE. Human sexual response. New York: Bantam; 1966.

55. Asimov J, Asimov I. How to enjoy writing: a book of aid and comfort. New York: Walker; 1987.

56. Groopman J, Hartzband P. Your medical mind: how to decide what is right for you. New York: Penguin; 2011.

57. Simpson E. For Doctor Howard Jones the work never ends. The Virginian-Pilot, 1 Dec 2014.

58. PSM V50 D093 Thomas Browne.jpg. This image is in the public domain because its copyright has expired. Available at: http://commons.wikimedia.org/wiki/File:PSM_V50_D093_Thomas_Browne.jpg.

59. Thomson A. Bodies of thought: science, religion, and the soul in the early enlightenment. New York: Oxford University Press; 2008.

60. Albert Schweitzer 1965.jpg. This file is licensed under the Creative Commons Attribution-Share Alike 3.0 Netherlands license.

61. Schweitzer A. The quest of the historical Jesus. London: A. & C. Black; 1910.

62. Collins F. The language of god: a scientist presents evidence for belief. New York: Simon & Schuster; 2006.

63. Isaacson W. Benjamin Franklin. New York: Simon & Schuster; 2003. p. 95.

64. Febvre L. The problem of unbelief in the 16th century: the religion of Rabelais. Cambridge, MA: Harvard College; 1982.

65. Yahr MD. A physician for all seasons: James Parkinson 1755–1824. Arch Neurol. 1978;35:185.

66. Tigertt WD. An annotated life of Egerton Yorrick Davis, MD: an intimate of Sir William Osler. J Hist Med Allied Sci. 1893;38:259.

67. Berra T. Charles Darwin: the concise story of an extraordinary man. Baltimore: Johns Hopkins University Press; 2008.

68. Connor CD. Jean Paul Marat: scientist and revolutionary. New York: Humanities Press; 1997.

69. Park M. Travels in the interior districts of Africa. London: Cassell; 1893.

70. Livingstone's 1871 Field Diary. David Livingstone Spectral Imaging Project. Livingstone Library, UCLA. Available at: http://livingstone.library.ucla.edu/1871diary/index.htm.

71. Sir Ronald Ross. Photograph. Wellcome V0028781.jpg. This file is licensed under the Creative Commons Attribution 4.0 International license. Available at: http://commons.wikimedia.org/wiki/File:Sir_Ronald_Ross._Photograph._Wellcome_V0028781.jpg.

72. Ross R. On some peculiar pigmented cells found in two mosquitoes fed on malarial blood. BMJ. 1897;2:1786.

73. Power NO. God of comics: Osamu Tezuka and the creation of post-world War II Manga. Jackson, MS: University Press of Mississippi; 2009.
74. Lau FH et al. Silas Weir Mitchell, MD: the physician who discovered causalgia. J Hand Surg Am. 2004;29:181.
75. Lee H. Virginia Woolf. London: Chatto & Windus; 1996.
76. Ellis HH. Sexual inversion. Available at: https://archive.org/details/cu31924013996958.
77. Ellis HH. Studies in the psychology of sex. First published in 1897. Available at: http://www.gutenberg.org/files/13610/13610-h/13610-h.htm.
78. Ellis HH. The task of social hygiene. Boston: Broughton Mifflin; 1912.
79. Havelock Ellis. New World Encyclopedia. Available at: http://www.newworldencyclopedia.org/entry/Havelock_Ellis.
80. Poppelwell R. Intelligence and imperial defense: British intelligence and the defense of the Indian empire. London: Routledge; 1995.
81. Cronin AJ. The citadel. Boston: Little, Brown; 1937.
82. Woodlief A. Lewis Thomas. Dictionary of literary biography, Vol. 275. Twentieth-Century American Nature Writers: Prose, 2003. Available from: http://www.vcu.edu/engweb/LewisThomas.htm/.
83. Kubler.jpg. This file has been released into the public domain by the copyright holder, its copyright has expired, or it is ineligible for copyright. This applies worldwide. Available at: http://psychology.wikia.com/wiki/File:Kubler.jpg.
84. Kübler-Ross E. The wheel of life. New York: Touchstone; 1998.
85. Gawande A. The cost conundrum—what a Texas town can teach us about health care. The New Yorker, 1 June 2009.
86. Pear R. Health care spending disparities stir a fight. The New York Times, 8 June 2009.
87. Maier T. Dr. Spock: an American life. New York: Basic Books; 2003.
88. Benjamin Spock 1968.jpg. This is a photo taken by Thomas R. Koeniges when working as a staff photographer of LOOK Magazine, and is part of the LOOK Magazine Photograph Collection at the Library of Congress. Their former owner, Cowles Communications, Inc., dedicated to the public all rights it owned to these images as an instrument of gift. http://commons.wikimedia.org/wiki/File:BenjaminSpock1968.jpg.
89. List of best-selling books. Available at: http://en.wikipedia.org/wiki/List_of_best-selling_books.

Chapter 9
What Writers Say About Writing

Writing is an intensely personal activity and one whose practitioners are generally articulate and insightful. Many of them have recorded memorable insights about writing, such as Truman Capote's distinction between "writing" and "typing," and Winston Churchill's description of writing a book: "Writing a book is an adventure. To begin with, it is a toy and an amusement; then it becomes a mistress, and then it becomes a master, and then a tyrant. The last phase is that just as you are about to be reconciled to your servitude, you kill the monster, and fling him out to the public" [1].

Here is what some other nonmedical writers have said about their craft [2]:

- "There is nothing to writing. All you do is sit down at a typewriter and bleed."
  – Ernest Hemingway
- "Lock up your libraries if you like; but there is no gate, no lock, no bolt that you can set upon the freedom of my mind."
  – Virginia Woolf, *A Room of One's Own*
- "You must stay drunk on writing so reality cannot destroy you."
  – Ray Bradbury, *Zen in the Art of Writing*
- "Writing is a socially acceptable form of schizophrenia."
  – E.L. Doctorow

Medical writing, as we have seen in prior chapters, is somewhat different than writing novels and short stories about general topics intended to be read by the public. This chapter tells what medical writers—some famous and some aspiring—have said about their writing (and their reading).

© Springer International Publishing Switzerland 2015
R.B. Taylor, *What Every Medical Writer Needs to Know*,
DOI 10.1007/978-3-319-20264-8_9

What Did Anton Chekhov Have to Say About Combining Medicine and Writing?

Russian physician and author Anton Pavlovich Chekhov (1860–1904) practiced medicine, but was not a huge financial success as a clinician (see Fig. 9.1). During his early days in medicine, Chekhov described his practice: "My medical practice keeps me busy … I have many friends and acquaintances and therefore not a few patients. Half of them I have to treat gratis, and the other half pay me three or five rubles for a visit …. I haven't made my fortune yet and I don't expect to make one soon" [4].

Later, Chekhov once wrote to a friend about his two loves [5]:

> "Medicine is my lawful wife, and literature is my mistress. When I get fed up with one, I spend the night with the other. Though it is irregular, it is less boring this way, and, besides, neither of them loses anything through my infidelity."

While we remember Chekhov's stories and plays, we sometimes overlook his 400-page work *The Island of Sakhalin*, a pioneering study of social medicine centered on a penal colony in Eastern Siberia considered Russia's "Devil's Island" [6]. Chekhov continued to write until tuberculosis caused his health to deteriorate. He died at age 44.

Fig. 9.1 Anton Pavlovich Chekhov, portrait by his brother Nikolay Chekhov [3] (this work is in the public domain)

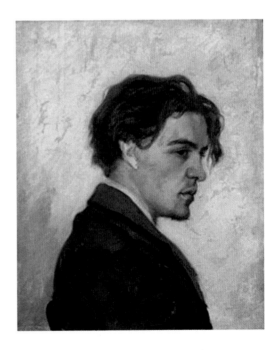

What Did Sir William Osler Say About Books and Reading?

Among his other exploits, Sir William Osler (1849–1919) wrote the first "big book" of the practice of medicine (see Fig. 9.2). Today there are other books of this scope in every generalist field and specialty, but these are all edited—compiled by a single editor or editorial team who recruit a "stable" of chapter authors who may number in the hundreds. In the years leading up to 1892, Osler wrote his epic work—*The Principles and Practice of Medicine*—all by himself.

In fact, writing the book consumed virtually all his spare hours, just at the time he was courting Grace Revere Gross, great-granddaughter of Revolutionary War hero Paul Revere and widow of a Philadelphia colleague. Grace suggested, firmly, that her suitor should finish his book before they married. In a tale that has become legend among Oslerian scholars, when Osler received his first copy of the book from the publisher, he tossed the heavy tome into Grace's lap and asked, "There, take the darn thing; now what are you going to do with the man?" Three months later they were married [8].

Osler was clearly a man who valued books as well as clinical learning. Here are two examples of what he believed about books, reading, and being a physician [9, 10]:

> "It is astonishing with how little reading a doctor can practice medicine, but it is not astonishing how badly he may do it."

AND

> "It is hard for me to speak of the value of libraries in terms that would not seem exaggerated. Books have been my delight these thirty years, and from them I have received incalculable benefits."

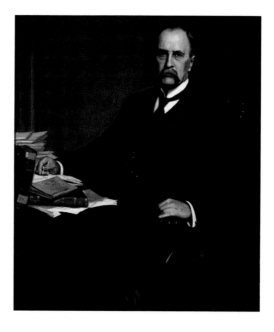

Fig. 9.2 Sir William Osler, author of the first comprehensive medical reference book, 1892 [7]

What Was Arthur E. Hertzler's Warning About the Urge to Write?

A rural physician who both made house calls and performed surgery, Arthur E. Hertzler (1870–1946) of Halstead, Kansas, penned and described it all in his best-selling book, *The Horse and Buggy Doctor*. The dust jacket of my copy of the book shows a physician riding in a horse-drawn buggy on a lonely country road. Here is what Hertzler said in the Preface about how he happened to write his book [11]:

> "Let this screed be a warning to all those who feel an urge to take up a pencil. It began innocently enough. My kid daughter, a trained nurse, being possessed of a small son, desired to know something of my early life so that she might institute prophylactic proceedings before it was too late. I chanced to tell a publisher friend, as an excuse for the delay in more important writing, what I was doing. At once he began his seductive procedures. The argument presented was that there should be a record of the old country doctor by one of the species."

What Did W. Somerset Maugham Tell About Being a Writer, the Best Training for a Writer, and the Three Basic Rules to Good Writing?

W. Somerset Maugham (1874–1965) successfully qualified as a physician and drove an ambulance in World War I (see Fig. 9.3). But he felt the lure of writing. Here is what he wrote about his apparently unanticipated success [13]:

> "I have never quite got over my astonishment at being a writer. There seems no reason for my having become one except an irresistible inclination."

Fig. 9.3 Sketch of W. Somerset Maugham by Edward Drantler [12]

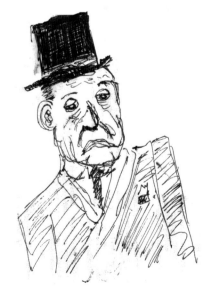

Maugham was well aware of the special advantage that his medical education afforded him in his writing career, and his writings often reflect characters with physical and emotional imperfections. He wrote the following about being both a physician and a writer [13]:

> "I do not know a better training for a writer than to spend some years in the medical profession. I suppose that you can learn a good deal about human nature in a solicitor's office; but there on the whole you have to deal with men in full control of themselves. They lie perhaps as much as they lie to the doctor, but they lie more consistently, and it may be that for the solicitor it is not so necessary to know the truth. The interests he deals with, besides, are usually material. He sees human nature from a specialized standpoint. But the doctor, especially the hospital doctor, sees it bare. Reticences can generally be undermined; very often there are none. Fear for the most part will shatter every defense; even vanity is unnerved by it. For most people have a furious itch to talk about themselves and are restrained only by the disinclination of others to listen. Reserve is an artificial quality that is developed in most of us but as the result of innumerable rebuffs. The doctor is discreet. It is his business to listen and no details are too intimate for his ears."

He was characterized by English writer George Orwell as the modern writer "whom I admire immensely for his power of telling a story straightforwardly and without frills." Clearly with tongue in cheek, Maugham tells the secret of good writing [13]:

> "There are three basic rules to good writing. Unfortunately, no one knows what they are."

How Did Alexander Fleming Describe the Impetus for His Book on Penicillin?

We remember Alexander Fleming (1881–1955) as the scientist who gave us penicillin, even though it was the serendipitous result of poor laboratory housekeeping (see Fig. 9.4). At least Fleming possessed what Louis Pasteur called the "prepared mind," and did not discard the culture dish contaminated with mold; instead he pondered how the presence of mold on the plate seemed to inhibit the growth of

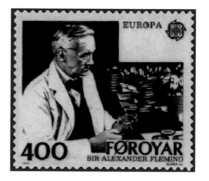

Fig. 9.4 Faroe Islands stamp showing Alexander Fleming with a disorderly collection of culture dishes. Photo credit: Postverk Føroya— Philatelic Office [14]

nearby bacterial colonies. The rest, as they say, is history, described in a book edited by Fleming himself. In the preface to his book, Fleming tells how the literary effort began [15]:

> "The publishers approached me to write a book for them on penicillin. This request I had to refuse for two very good reasons: first I had too many commitments to spare the time to do justice to the book, and secondly it would have been impossible for me, a laboratory worker, to place penicillin therapy in its proper perspective relative to other forms of medical and surgical treatment in a great variety of conditions."

Despite his stated initial reluctance, Fleming went on to produce a book titled *Penicillin: Its Practical Application*. It was an edited volume, with Fleming writing the introductory chapter followed by contributions by more than two dozen scientists and clinicians. I was intrigued by a final chapter titled "Penicillin and the General Practitioner," in which the author, on page 350, describes "penicillin injections every 3 hours for 7 or more days ..."

Fleming's prefatory comments are significant to medical writers in two ways. First of all, the most successful—that is, robust sales—books are generally not proposed by the prospective authors/editors, but are suggested by the publisher. Secondly, despite the fact that I really prefer to write my books with no coauthors and with a "voice," clinical science and practice have evolved in complexity to the point that production of an authoritative reference book generally is a team effort involving multiple contributors.

How Did William Carlos Williams Describe His Dual Careers in Medicine and Writing?

William Carlos Williams (1883–1963) both practicing physician and award-winning poet once remarked, "I think all writing is a disease. You can't stop it" (see Fig. 9.5). He tried to make his works reflect the ordinary people he encountered every day, including the events they experienced and sometimes even how they spoke. Describing one poem he had written, he explained [17]:

> "The poem springs from the half-spoken words of such patients as the physician sees from day to day."

Not unlike W. Somerset Maugham (above), Williams was keenly aware of how much his active medical practice and daily contact with patients brought to his writing [17]:

> "That is why as a writer I have never felt that medicine interfered with me but rather that it was my very food and drink, the very thing which made it possible for me to write. Was I not interested in man? There the thing was, right in front of me. I could touch it, smell it. It was myself, naked, just as it was, without a lie telling itself to me in its own terms. Oh, I knew it wasn't for the most part giving me anything very profound, but it was giving me terms, basic terms with which I could spell out matters as profound as I cared to think of."

Fig. 9.5 Passport photograph of American poet and medical doctor William Carlos Williams, 1921. Image courtesy of the Beinecke Rare Book & Manuscript Library, Yale University [16]

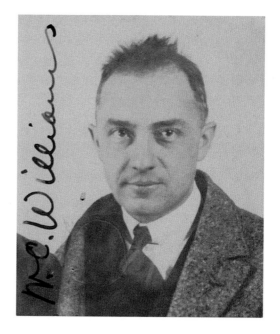

How Did Morris Fishbein Describe the Manner in Which Medical Writers Sometimes Agonize Over Their Works?

Morris Fishbein (1889–1976) was an American physician who was the editor in chief of the *Journal of the American Medical Association* (JAMA) from 1924 to 1950. He also wrote several books, including *The Medical Follies: An Analysis of the Foibles of Some Healing Cults, Including Osteopathy, Homeopathy, Chiropractic, and The Electronic Reactions of Abrams, with Essays on the Anti-Vivisectionists, Health Legislation, Physical Culture, Birth Control, and Rejuvenation* [18]. He also wrote a book for medical writers: *Medical Writing: The Technic and the Art*. In the Introduction to the third edition of the Medical Writing book, Fishbein observed metaphorically [19]:

> "Increasing organization in the field of medicine, as in every other field of human endeavor, has raised the level of contributions to medical literature. Far too often, however, physicians still prepare their contributions with a striving and agony and delay comparable to the delivery of human progeny by one untutored in the refinement of obstetrics."

What Sort of Reading Did Félix Martí-Ibáñez Recommend for Those Who Wanted to Understand the Medical Thinking of Some Period in History?

Spanish-American physician, writer, and publisher Félix Martí-Ibáñez (1911–1972) was founding editor of *MD Magazine*, a position he held from 1957 until his death in 1972. He also served as Professor of the History Of Medicine at New York Medical College. He once wrote of the importance of clear communication [20]:

> "The physician today has a special obligation: to speak and write about what he sees and knows, and to do so clearly, harmoniously, and euphonically, as he can."

In this same book, Martí-Ibáñez writes of how he believes a reader can best step back into the history of medicine:

> "If I were asked what sort of documents I would choose to comprehend better the medical history of any one period, I would choose not the biographies of the great scientists, not even an enumeration of the great medical discoveries in that period; I would choose a representative clinical case history scribbled by a physician at the bedside of his patient. For such a humble document indeed affords a live, meaningful summary of the clinical know-how of an age, archetypically represented in the practical wisdom of a general practitioner. No other document can throw as much light on the evolution of medical knowledge through the centuries as the ordinary clinical case history."

What Was Wilder Penfield's Opinion of the Influence of Medical Textbooks?

I first came to know Wilder Penfield (1861–1976) as the author of *The Torch*, a fictionalized account of the life of Hippocrates on the island of Kos [21]. But the author was also an internationally renowned neurosurgeon, a pioneer in mapping the cortices of the brain, and recipient of the 1960 Lister Medal to acknowledge his advancement of surgical science. Penfield's comments quoted below raise issues pertinent for medicine's future as we think about the many guidelines for practice currently being promulgated [22]:

> "The Egyptians made a mistake. They wrote textbooks, the hermetic books. They made another and more serious mistake, and that was to believe that the textbooks were correct. So they forbid physicians, at peril of their lives, to depart in any way from the treatment prescribed in the hermetic books. It was a remarkable experiment … The experiment demonstrated that standardization can halt advance but it does not in any way hinder retrogression."

Who Did Physician-Author Ferrol Sams Identify as His Audience?

American physician-writer Ferrol Sams (1922–2013) and his physician wife, Helen, spent their medical careers practicing in Fayette County, Georgia. Drawing strongly on the southern traditions of his life, Sams was the author of eight books, including

Run with the Horsemen (1982) and *When All the World Was Young* (1992). In a recorded interview with the Georgia Writers Hall of Fame on October 1, 2012, Sams said: "Reading is the first door that opens to the outside world, for anybody" [23].

Some criticized the "folksy" nature of his stories. But in the interview noted above, Sams was asked whom he wrote for. He gave a one-word answer [23]:

"Myself"

He went on to add [23]:

"If you lose your sense of awe, or if you lose your sense of the ridiculous, you've fallen into a terrible pit. The only thing that's worse is never to have had either."

And:

"A good editor's job is to protect an author from himself, from falling in love with a favorite line."

How Does Richard Selzer Explain Why Surgeons Write?

Richard Selzer (1928–) is an American surgeon and author, born in Troy, New York. In addition to a busy practice, Selzer wrote a number of popular books, including *Mortal Lessons: Notes on the Art of Surgery* (1976), *Confessions of a Knife* (1979), and his autobiographical *Down from Troy: A Doctor Comes of Age* (1992).

Writing in *Mortal Lessons: Notes on the Art of Surgery*, Selzer reflects [24]:

"Someone asks me why a surgeon would write. Why, when the shelves area already too full? They sag under the dead weight of books. To add a single adverb is to risk exceeding the strength of the boards."

Later in the page he gives us an answer:

"It (i.e. writing) is to search for some meaning in the ritual of surgery, which is at once murderous, painful, healing, and full of love …"

Selzer was sued for alleged malpractice, the claim filed 2 years after the surgeon retired from active practice. One way Selzer coped with this blow was to write about it. In an article published in the *New York Times*, he describes his "anorexia, insomnia and a sense of bereavement as though, 50 years later, I am once again grieving for my father." In the end, the case was withdrawn; Selzer won, but not without great anguish during the trial, as he describes in his narrative, *Trial and Tribulation* [25].

Why Does Robin Cook Believe His Books Are Popular?

Robin Cook (1940–) writes medical thrillers (see Fig. 9.6). He also has a penchant for short, often one-word, titles. Many of us have spent leisure hours reading *Coma* (1977), *Outbreak* (1887), *Terminal* (1993), and *Cell* (2014). Cook once quipped: "I joke that if my books stop selling, I can always fall back on brain surgery" [27].

Fig. 9.6 American
medical writer Robin
Cook, 2008. Photo credit:
Patryk Korzeniecki [26]

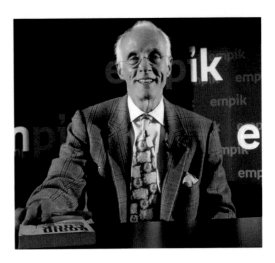

In an interview with Jay McDonald, Cook explained the universal appeal of his novels [27]:

> "The main reason is, we all realize we are at risk. We're all going to be patients sometime."
> "You can write about great white sharks or haunted houses, and you can say I'm not going into the ocean or I'm not going in haunted houses, but you can't say you're not going to go into a hospital."

How Does Khaled Hosseini Begin Work on a Book?

The Kite Runner was the first novel by Afghan-born American physician Khaled Hosseini (1965–), published in 2003. The book describes the life of a boy living in Afghanistan following the Russian invasion. Subsequently the author wrote *A Thousand Splendid Suns* (2007) and *And the Mountains Echoed* (2013). Like Chekhov before him, Hosseini reflects: "Medicine was an arranged marriage, writing is my mistress" [28].

In a 2013 interview reported by David Miller, the author tells how he started work on his latest novel [28]:

> "To doodle with words. First a very vivid image of a little radio-flyer red wagon, the one like we all grew up on. Doodling … traveling across a desert. Doodling … inside of it was this cute little girl, maybe about three. Then doodling a few paces back, a little boy about ten. This image was just so startling in how vivid and clear it was, it became very clear that the little girl and the boy were brother and sister and they had this very deep and powerful bond, and loved each other and they were headed to Kabul with their father."

What Do Some Professional Medical Writers Have to Say About Medical Writing?

The comments above are, for the most part, by physician-writers who tell stories, and not by *professional medical writers,* the ones who write research protocols, advertising copy, new drug submissions, newspaper columns, and all the other work products that call for someone who is knowledgeable about the topic and is a skilled wordsmith. These writers may not see their names in print, but they are vitally important to the companies or the academic medical centers that employ them. Or perhaps the person is a freelance writer. You may never have heard of the medical writers quoted below, but it is just possible that their work might have influenced your health care:

"Medical writing is a diverse field, comprising publications and educational, promotional, and regulatory writing. Each of these domains includes numerous sub-genres and a vast and ever-expanding range of therapeutic areas. Even so, successful medical writers share traits in common. These include a love of language, strong attention to detail, high ethical standards, the tenacity to see a project through, the desire to continually learn about science and medicine, the ability to gracefully receive and implement feedback, and the resilience and self-discipline to work for long hours in relative isolation." (Amy Karon) [29]

"I looked for a career offering plenty of variety, but which gave me the opportunity to do more of the thing that I enjoyed doing most: medical writing." (Ryan Woodrow) [30]

"I would recommend a career in medical writing to anyone who wants to combine their passion for learning about new science and medicine with their enjoyment of writing." (Anon. Quoted by Ryan Woodrow) [30]

"Medical writing is different from other types of professional writing because it incorporates knowledge, methods, and terminology from a variety of fields. For instance, biostatistics, journalism, medicine, English, public health, and pharmacy are fields that most medical writers tend to consult regularly." (Brent Ardaugh) [31]

"After a DPhil and five years post-doctoral research I found that I had gradually come to enjoy communicating biomedical science much more than actually doing research." (Martin Callaghan) [32]

Is There One Saying About Medical Writing That Seems to Pull It All Together?

John Shaw Billings (1838–1913), the physician who updated the Library of the Office of the Surgeon General of the Army, now known as the National Library of Medicine, wrote on a variety of topics. Among his published works are *Medical Museums* (1888), *National Medical Dictionary* (1889), and *Physiological Aspects of the Liquor Problem* (1903) (see Fig. 9.7). Here is his advice about writing a medical paper (or, for that matter, a book chapter or book) [34]:

"First have something to say, 2nd say it, 3rd stop when you have said it, and finally give it an accurate title."

Fig. 9.7 Cabinet card
image of American
surgeon and librarian John
Shaw Billings. Source:
Harvard Theater
Collection, Harvard
University [33]

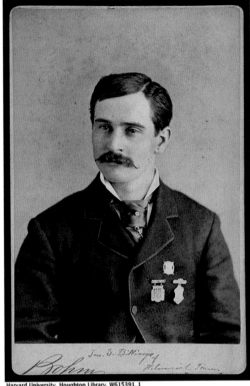

Harvard University, Houghton Library, W615391_1

References

1. Winston Churchill quotes. Available at: http://thinkexist.com/quotation/writing_a_book_is_
   an_adventure-to_begin_with-it/15860.html.
2. Quotes about writing. Available at: http://www.goodreads.com/quotes/tag/writing.
3. Chehov Anton by Nikolay Chekhov.jpg. This work is in the public domain in the United
   States, and those countries with a copyright term of life of the author plus 100 years or less.
   Available at: http://en.wikipedia.org/wiki/File:Chehov_anton_by_nikolay_chekhov.jpg.
4. Magarshack D. Chekhov—a life. Westport, CT: Greenwood Press; 1970.
5. Letter to Alexei Suvorin, 11 Sept 1888. In: Letters of Anton Chekhov to his family and friends,
   trans. Garnett C. Available at: http://www.gutenberg.org/files/6408/6408-h/6408-h.htm.
6. Carter R, Anton P. Chekhov, MD (1860–1904): dual medical and literary careers. Ann Thorac
   Surg. 1996;61:1557.
7. Sir William Osler.jpg. This work is in the public domain. Available at: http://commons.wiki-
   media.org/wiki/File:Sir_William_Osler.jpg.
8. Osler and Grace visit Tracadie. Osler Libr Newsl. 2008;110:1.
9. Osler W. Aphorisms. In: Reynolds R et al., editors. On doctoring. New York: Simon &
   Schuster; 1991. p. 30.
10. Osler W. In: Silverman ME et al., editors. The quotable Osler. Philadelphia: American Collage
    of Physicians; 2003, p. 198.

11. Hertzler AE. The horse and buggy doctor. New York: Harper Brothers; 1938. Preface.
12. Maugham.png. This file is licensed under the Creative Commons Attribution-Share Alike 3.0 Unported license. Available at: http://commons.wikimedia.org/wiki/File:Maugham.png.
13. Maugham WS. The summing up. New York: Doubleday, Doran; 1938.
14. Faroe stamp 079 europe (fleming).jpg. Engraver: Czesław Słania. Printing: National Bank of Finland, Helsingfors. This file has been released into the public domain by its copyright holder, Postverk Føroya—Philatelic Office. Available at: http://commons.wikimedia.org/wiki/File:Faroe_stamp_079_europe_(fleming).jpg.
15. Fleming A. Penicillin: its practical application. Philadelphia: Blakiston; 1946. Preface.
16. William Carlos Williams passport photograph 1921.jpg. This work is in the public domain in the United States because it is a work prepared by an officer or employee of the United States Government as part of that person's official duties under the terms of Title 17, Chapter 1, Section 105 of the US Code. Available at: http://commons.wikimedia.org/wiki/File:William_Carlos_Williams_passport_photograph_1921.jpg.
17. Williams WC. The practice. In: The autobiography of William Carlos Williams. New York: New Directions; 1967.
18. Fishbein M. The medical follies: an analysis of the foibles of some healing cults, including osteopathy, homeopathy, chiropractic, and the electronic reactions of Abrams, with essays on the anti-vivisectionists, health legislation, physical culture, birth control, and rejuvenation. New York: Boni & Liveright; 1925.
19. Fishbein M. Medical writing: the technic and the art. 3rd ed. New York: Blakiston; 1957.
20. Martí-Ibáñez F. Men, molds, and history. New York: MD Publications; 1958.
21. Penfield W. The torch. Boston: Little, Brown; 1960.
22. Penfield W. The second career. Boston: Little, Brown; 1963.
23. Interview with Ferrol Sams. Georgia Writers Hall of Fame Interview: 1 Oct 2012. Available at: https://www.youtube.com/watch?v=aex99Qwy0Cw.
24. Selzer R. Mortal lessons: notes on the art of surgery. New York: Simon & Schuster; 1974, p. 15.
25. Selzer R. Trial and tribulation. The New York Times, 23 Sept 1990. Available at: http://www.nytimes.com/1990/09/23/magazine/trial-and-tribulation.html?src=pm&pagewanted=1.
26. Robin Cook in Warsaw Poland 2008.jpg. This file is licensed under the Creative Commons Attribution-Share Alike 3.0 Unported license. Available at http://commons.wikimedia.org/wiki/File:Robin_Cook_in_Warsaw_Poland_2008.jpg.
27. McDonald J. Robin Cook. In: BookPage. Available at: http://bookpage.com/interviews/8111-robin-cook#.VHdAUKTF9fU.
28. Miller D. Khaled Hosseini author of Kite Runner talks about his mistress: writing. Loveland Magazine, 7 June 2013. Available at: http://www.lovelandmagazine.com/2013/06/khaled-hosseni-talks-about-his-mistress-writing.html.
29. Karon A. Tips for new medical writers. Karon Medical Writing. Available at: http://amykaron.com/tips-for-new-medical-writers/.
30. Woodrow R. Been there, done it, got the T-shirt. The life of a medical writer. Available at: http://www.slideshare.net/woodrowr/the-life-of-a-medical-writer-tips-for-people-considering-a-medical-writing-career.
31. Ardaugh B. Online Writing Lab. Purdue University Owl. Available at: https://owl.english.purdue.edu/owl/resource/732/01/.
32. Callaghan M. Comments: MedComms. Available at: http://www.medcommsnetworking.co.uk/docs/quotes_newbies.pdf.
33. Harvard Theater Collection—JS Billings TCS 1.2489.jpg. This image (or other media file) is in the public domain because its copyright has expired. Available at: http://commons.wikimedia.org/wiki/File:Harvard_Theatre_Collection_-_J_S_Billings_TCS_1.2489.jpg.
34. Billings JS. Quoted in: Strauss MB. Familiar medical quotations. Boston: Little, Brown; 1968.

Chapter 10
A Writer's Attic

A book of this type needs a miscellaneous chapter—a place to put all the odd pieces that don't fit the previous chapter headings, an attic to hold all the gee-whiz things just too good to discard. This is that chapter.

What Was America's First and Oldest Medical Journal?

This is a trick question. The *first* medical journal in America was *The Medical Repository*, debuting in print in 1797. There were three original coeditors: Elihu H. Smith, Samuel L. Mitchill, and Edward Miller. T & J Swords, affiliated with Columbia College in New York City, was the printer. Although there were some interruptions, *The Medical Repository* continued to be published until 1824 [1].

America's *oldest* medical journal in continuous publication is the *New England Journal of Medicine* (NEJM), which began in Boston in 1812 as the *New England Journal of Medicine and Surgery and the Collateral Branches of Medical Science* (see Fig. 10.1). John Collins Warren and James Jackson were the founding editors. In 1828, the publication became the *Boston Medical and Surgical Journal*. Then in 1921, the Massachusetts Medical Society, for the grand sum on $1, purchased the journal, and renamed it the *New England Journal of Medicine* [3].

In a sense, the earliest American journals were emulating medical journals that had existed in Europe for a century. Generally regarded as the first medical journal in the Western World, *Le Journal des Sçavans* was first published in France in 1665, followed later that year in England by *Philosophical Transactions* [4].

It didn't take long for medical and scientific journals to proliferate. At the beginning of the nineteenth century there were approximately 30 scientific journals, and a hundred years later the number had grown to more than 700 publications for the medical and research community.

© Springer International Publishing Switzerland 2015
R.B. Taylor, *What Every Medical Writer Needs to Know*,
DOI 10.1007/978-3-319-20264-8_10

THE

NEW ENGLAND JOURNAL

OF

MEDICINE AND SURGERY.

| Vol. 1.] | JANUARY, 1812. | [No. I. |

REMARKS ON ANGINA PECTORIS.

BY JOHN WARREN, M. D.

In our inquiries into any particular subject of Medicine, our labours will generally be shortened and directed to their proper objects, by a knowledge of preceding discoveries.

When Dr. Heberden, in the London Medical Transactions, first described a disease under the name of Angina Pectoris, so little had it attracted the attention of physicians, that much surprise was excited by the communication. From the most striking and distressing symptoms, with which it was attended, pain and stricture about the breast, it received from him its denomination ; and he soon after published farther remarks on this subject, with the history of a case and appearances on dissection.

That all the cases which this author had noticed as accompanied with affections of *a somewhat similar nature,* were instances of true Angina Pectoris, is by no means probable ; for not less than one hundred of those were supposed by him to have fallen under his observation. Of those, three only were women, one a boy ; all the rest were men, and about the age of fifty.

In the same work were communicated some observations on this disease made by Dr. Wall, who likewise added a case of dissection.

Dr. Fothergill, in the fifth volume of the London Medical Observations and Inquiries, 1774, published his remarks upon An-

VOL. I.   1

What Was the Most Remarkable Feat of Medical Writing (in More or Less Modern Times) and What Is Also Remarkable About the Title?

My vote would be for *The Principles and Practice of Medicine*, written single-handedly by Sir William Osler and published in 1892. In my opinion, it was the *"War and Peace"* of medical writing, of epic scope (and heft). Osler's book survived through many editions until 2001, although it eventually became an edited volume with many contributors [5]. A later competitor was the *Cecil Textbook of Medicine*, edited by Russell Cecil, MD, and initially published in 1927. But Cecil relied on many contributors to accomplish what Osler had done on his own. I recently noted a copy of Osler's first edition offered for sale on line for only $4750 [6].

As an aside, Osler was not the first to use the title *The Principles and Practice of Medicine*. That title was previously that of a book by English physician and author John Elliotson, first published in England in 1839 (see Fig. 10.2). Elliotson was a member of the Royal College of Physicians, a friend of Charles Dickens, and a strong advocate of mesmerism [8]. Is borrowing a title of a book published a half century before a breech of ethics? The US copyright laws think not, unless there is "a signifi-cant amount of original expression," a phrase which, like "fair use" (of borrowed material), is not clearly defined. Today, if I wanted to title my next book using the same words as Elliotson and Osler, I could do so with reasonable confidence, but not if my next book were titled, for instance, *The Lord of the Rings* or *The Da Vinci Code*, both of which seem to have a good deal of "original expression" [9].

Has There Been a Recent Change of Focus in Medical Journals?

The change has been subtle, and I had not noticed the shift in emphasis until I read the article by cardiologist Wes Fisher appearing on the website Kevinmd.com/blog. The title of Fisher's article tells it all: "Medical Journals Are Shifting From Science to Politics" [10].

The author uses as his example the NEJM, considered by the *New York Times* to be the "most prestigious" of all medical journals [11]. He compares articles from his latest issue of the NEJM to those printed a decade before, finding a remarkable shift from an emphasis on scientific discoveries to a focus on sociopolitical topics.

This prompted me to look at the Table of Contents of my recent issues of NEJM and the *Journal of the American Medical Association* (JAMA). I found some purely scientific reports on the transfusion threshold in septic shock (NEJM), glycemic control in type I diabetes (NEJM), and comparative weight loss among named diet programs (JAMA), all containing information important to me as a generalist physician.

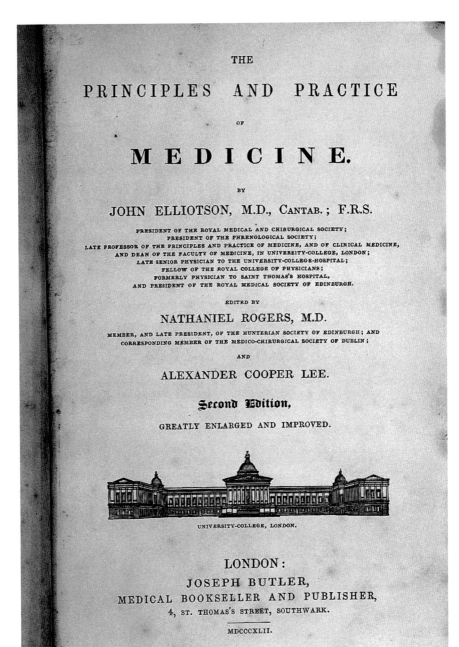

Fig. 10.2 Title page of *The Principles and Practice of Medicine, 2nd edition*, by John Elliotson, 1842, published a half century before Olser's book of the same title [7]

But in my same journals I encountered articles on calorie labeling in restaurants, barriers to physician reimbursement, life insurers having access to genetic results, diversity in medical education, hospital relationships with direct-to-consumer screening companies, government regulation of portion size, the blockade of Medicaid, and the inevitable debates about the Affordable Care Act.

Why the change? Certainly the shifting focus reflects the increasing impact of economics and regulations on the process and outcome of health care. Any health care system is profoundly influenced by what doctors and other professionals are allowed to do and how they are paid for doing it. On all of these issues and more, the sociopolitical articles in our most influential "scientific" journals inevitably reflect a viewpoint. That is what op-ed articles do. But who determines what is published and the viewpoint reflected?

And, for those involved in treating actual sick patients, every political opinion article printed means another clinical trial report not published and read by those in practice. For medical writers, it is one more op-ed piece and one less research report.

What Is an "Authorism" and Is This Something Medical Writers Ever Do?

In the Introduction to this chapter I alerted you that it represented a potpourri. Hence I am going to shift from history and politics to a lighter topic: made-up words.

An "authorism" is a new word created, and sometimes championed, by an author. Authorisms are invented words that catch on because they seem to fill a need. Otherwise they don't survive. Perhaps I am being restrictive, but I don't consider a new word an authorism unless the creator of the term can be identified.

The word authorism seems itself, to be an authorism, the brainchild of Paul Dickson, who describes a number of such neologisms in his 2014 book appropriately titled *Authorisms: Words Wrought by Writers* [12]. One of the best known of these is the word "serendipity," first used by Horace Walpole in a 1754 letter to his friend Horace Mann, alluding to the Persian folk tale of "The Three Princes of Serendip" (now called Sri Lanka). The princely trio had the facility of repeatedly making chance but happy discoveries. Dickson goes on to describe the words "pandemonium" (John Milton), "chortle" (Lewis Carroll), and "butterfingers" (Charles Dickens) as authorisms. My favorite: American scholar H.L. Menken, aka "the sage of Baltimore," created the term ecdysiast, based on the word "ecdysis," i.e., the process of shedding old skin, molting. This new word was his gift to famous striptease artist Gypsy Rose Lee (immortalized in the movie *Gypsy*), who sought a more elegant term to describe her role on stage [13]. The creation of the verb "neologize" has been attributed to President Thomas Jefferson, along with some 100 other words such as "pedicure" and "indecipherable" [14].

What About Medical Authorisms?

- **Ambidextrous and others**: In the seventeenth century, Sir Thomas Browne, author of *Religio Medici* (The Religion of a Physician), introduced dozens of new terms, many of them part of our current medical vocabulary. Among them are the words ambidextrous, ascetic, locomotion, prostate, and suicide [15, 16].
- **Vaccinate**: In 1796 Edward Jenner was the first to use the word "vaccinate," a very reasonable term considering that the material he used to protect humans from smallpox came from a cow (*vacca* in Latin).
- *Streptococcus* **and** *Staphylococcus*: In the mid-nineteenth century, the word "*Streptococcus*" was coined by Viennese physician Albert Theodor Billroth, based on Latin and Greek roots and describing bacteria seen in "chains." Billroth's name is part of the today's surgical lexicon, used to describe a gastric reconstruction procedure (see Fig. 10.3). About this same time, Scottish surgeon and scientist Alexander Ogston gave us a new word, "*Staphylococcus*," coming from similar roots, and identifying bacteria seen occurring in clusters under the microscope [16].
- **Phantom limb**: The phenomenon of perceiving sensation, sometimes including pain, following amputation of a limb had been known as early as the time of Ambroise Paré in the sixteenth century, but it was not until 1871 that American physician and writer Silas Weir Mitchell created the authorism "phantom limb" [18].
- **Anesthesia**: William T.G. Morton introduced us to ether insensitivity to pain, but Oliver Wendell Holmes, Sr. gave us the word "anesthesia" [19].

Fig. 10.3 Albert Theodor Billroth, considered by some to be the father of modern abdominal surgery [17]

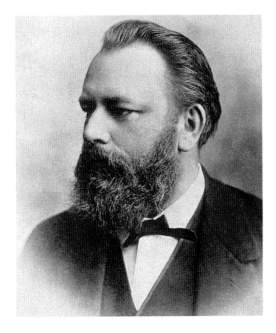

- **Microalbuminuria**: In 1964, Harry Keen, Professor of Metabolism at Saint Guy's Medical School in London, introduced the word "microalbuminuria," describing small amounts of albumin in the urine [20].
- **Gomer**: In his satirical description of hospital life, *The House of God*, published in 1978, psychiatrist Steven Bergman, pseudonymously writing as Samuel Shem, MD, gave us the medical slang word gomer, to describe a patient who "has lost— often through age—what goes into being a human being." Gomer is, in fact, an acronym for "Get outta my emergency room," and thus probably should be in all capitals—i.e., GOMER—just like SCUBA and AIDS. Two of the Laws of The House of God are [21]:

  1. Gomers don't die; and
  2. Gomers go to ground.

- **Diabesity**: "Diabesity," the combination of diabetes and obesity, entered our vocabulary with the publication of the book by Dr. Francine Kaufman titled *Diabesity: The Obesity-Diabetes Epidemic That Threatens America—And What We Must Do to Stop It* [22]. A current Google search of the word "diabesity" yielded several dozen sites; Kaufman's neologism seems to have "stuck."
- **Singularity**: Also in 2005, futurist author Ray Kurzweil coined the term "singularity" to describe the time when humans and computers will merge as one through the addition of technological advances, such as tiny nanobots, to our brain function [23].
- **iPatient**: In 2008, American physician Abraham Verghese gave us the freshly minted word "iPatient," to describe the virtual patient discussed by students and residents while viewing online laboratory reports "in the bunker while the real patients keep the beds warm and ensure that the folders bearing their names stay alive on the computer" [24].

Not all attempts at medial authorism are successful. Some are proposed, but never really catch the fancy of the medical writing community. Consider the following:

- **Balneation and others**: Sir Thomas Browne, mentioned above, proposed some words that aren't often encountered today: "balneation" (bathing), "moratin" (a delay), and "pistillation" (to grind with a pestle) [15].
- **Homogenic**: In Chap. 8, I told of British physician-author Havelock Ellis who wrote on homosexuality, but deplored the term, preferring the word "homogenic." Today we sometimes use the word "homophobic," but "homogenic" today has another meaning entirely. It is used in genetics to mean "having only one alternative form, or one allele, of a gene or genes" [25].
- **Journalology**: The term "journalology" is the brainchild of former *British Medical Journal* editor Stephen Lock [26]. The word describes the use of biometrics to evaluate journals, and has to do with the impact factor, described in Chap. 3. The word "journalology", however, has no entry in Dictionary.com, and I can't say I have ever heard it used in conversation.
- **Neosyndrome**: Just below, I use this term. I just made it up. Time will tell if anyone uses the word again.

What Is the Role of the Neosyndrome?

This, the word "neosyndrome," is a neologism, an authorism I created just for fun. I could not find it in any dictionary, my MS Word Spellchecker rejects it, and a Google search comes up empty. It designates a newly described syndrome, which may be a recently recognized constellation of symptoms and signs, or perhaps a descriptive title for a behavioral or physical manifestation we all know. Some neosyndrome names involve place names, or activities, or even the names of patients. Some involve irony and wicked wit.

- **Little League pitcher's elbow and more**: Among the diseases named for activities are "little pitcher's elbow," "silo-filler disease," "gamekeeper thumb," "tennis elbow," and "welder's conjunctivitis." "Saturday night paralysis" occurs when an alcohol sedated individual sleeps with an arm over the armrest of a chair or the back of a park bench, sustaining a radial nerve palsy. When garment workers return after a weekend to a factory with the air laden with cotton dust, they may suffer "Monday morning asthma." Then there is the "Sleeping Beauty syndrome" (a pathologic sleep disturbance). Sometime, somewhere, someone thought up all these descriptors. All were once freshly described neosyndromes.
- **Christmas disease**: In 1952, Biggs et al. told of a new type of bleeding disorder—Christmas disease—named for the first patient described with the hematologic abnormality, Stephen Christmas [27]. Were editors indulging their sense of humor when the article appeared in the *British Medical Journal* Christmas issue? The eponymous title of the disease has endured. But would it have been so if the index case had been John Jones or Mary Smith?
- **Alice in Wonderland syndrome**: The term "Alice in Wonderland" syndrome describes perceived alterations in body image sometimes seen with migraine or epilepsy; it was first used medically in 1955 by British psychiatrist John Todd, alluding to the well-known Lewis Carroll book *Alice's Adventures in Wonderland* [28] (see Fig. 10.4).

Fig. 10.4 In the "Alice in Wonderland" syndrome, the patient experiences distorted perceptions of body images [29]

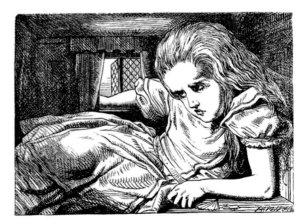

- **The Ulysses syndrome**: We have an entire universe of iatrogenic syndromes caused by therapeutic misadventures. The Ulysses syndrome, first described by Rang in 1972, is different. It is a side effect of investigation, and also might be identified as the "laboratory error syndrome" or the "top/bottom of the bell curve syndrome." The non-disease begins with the discovery of an unanticipated abnormality on a laboratory panel or roentgenogram. This prompts a return visit to the doctor, who dispatches the healthy patient on an odyssey of unnecessary testing, imaging, and perhaps scoping. The most serious risk of being the victim of the Ulysses syndrome is not the wasted time and money, but the very real possibility that the investigation might culminate in needless therapy or even invasive surgery [30].
- **Legionnaires' disease**: Legionnaires' disease was so named because the index cases were American Legion members all staying in the Bellevue-Stratford Hotel on Broad Street in Philadelphia in July 1976. The disease, of course, has no other connection with this respected veteran's organization, and I suspect its members wish the new disease had been named something else, perhaps the Bellevue-Stratford disease. But it may be too late to call it Philadelphia disease.
- **Kabuki syndrome**: "Kabuki syndrome," described by Kuroki in 1981, takes its name from the facial similarity of patients to the makeup of actors in traditional Japanese Kabuki Theater. Those afflicted have large ears, elongated palpebral fissures, a depressed tip of the nose, skeletal abnormalities, and mental retardation [31].
- **SARS**: In 2003, we witnessed the emergence of severe acute respiratory syndrome (SARS), which began in China, and, thanks to the miracle of modern air travel, eventually killed 775 persons in 37 countries. The name given hastily to the manifestations—severe acute respiratory syndrome—was not especially inventive, or even descriptive of the geographic or other locus of origin.

  In April 2014 the USA recognized its first case of another acute pulmonary disease, named the Middle Eastern respiratory syndrome (MERS) [32]. The infected individual had recently returned home to Munster, Indiana, from Saudi Arabia. Both SARS and MERS are neosyndromes, as was the acquired immunodeficiency syndrome (AIDS) in the 1980s.
- *Borrelia miyamotoi* **disease**: Lyme disease, caused by *Borrelia burgdorferi*, is named for Lyme, Connecticut, where a cluster of cases occurred in 1975. Now we have a new disease, caused by a cousin of *B. burgdorferi* named *B. miyamotoi*, detected first in Connecticut and subsequently found to be spread by all the same tick species that are the vectors for Lyme disease [33]. "*Borrelia miyamotoi* disease" is much too cumbersome a title for continued use, and so this new disease is a naming opportunity for someone.
- **Philadelphia syndrome**: In searching for neosyndromes, I came to the 2013 description of a mystery ailment affecting chiefly young women in the Philadelphia area, characterized by sudden personality changes, uncontrolled movements, and seizures. Physicians report, "It is like your brain is on fire" [34]. Will this entity, in time, come to be known as "Philadelphia syndrome?"

- **PCHD**: In the wicked wit category is "political correctness hyperactivity disorder (PCHD)," a neosyndrome concept promulgated by Martin in a letter to the editor in the *Wall Street Journal* describing America's current state of political affairs [35]. The author writes, "What we have before us is a postmodern magisterium of secular doctrine, affected with political correctness hyperactivity disorder (PCHD) and fueled by a utopian ambition that see no limits to its quest for power in the guise of public service."

I Just Received an Unsolicited E-mail Invitation to Edit a New Medical Reference Book. I Have Never Heard of the Publisher Before. Would This Be a Good Career Move?

In Chap. 5 I described predatory publishers soliciting manuscripts for open-access journals whose chief goal was to extract publication fees from authors of scientific papers. There is a related online scheme to rob you of something more valuable than a few dollars—your reputation in the scientific community. What they want is your good name.

Recently I also received an "out-of-the-blue," e-mail request to edit an ebook titled *Current Developments in Stroke*. This would seem to be a great honor. Finally someone recognizes my many valued contributions to the medical literature. Even though my "plate" is full, who could refuse such an opportunity? I would receive a 5 % royalty on sales, and all I would have to do is to "solicit chapter contributions from active, eminent scientists, largely from developed countries, with a focus on an important theme of current interest" [36]. I would then presumably correct all errors, arrange the chapters in an orderly folder on my computer, and send them on to the publisher. Did I mention that this proposal describes not a single work, but an entire ebook series?

My first hint of something amiss was the topic proposed. I have written more that 30 medical books and some 200 published papers, including a few articles on the topic of migraine headache. But I am certainly not an expert on stroke, nor am I a "scientist." Thus, despite my editing experience, I seemed an odd choice to edit a work on stroke.

Then there was the publisher, which I will not name here. A quick Google check revealed that this publisher has its home offices in Sharjah, one of the emirates of the United Arab Emirates, and that it publishes more than 100 "scientific" journals and offers a number of free-to-view online publications. Perhaps nothing too alarming so far. But the publisher has its critics. A Wikipedia search on June 1, 2014, cites reports of this same publisher "spamming scientists to become a member of the editorial boards of its journals," and having "exploited the Open Access model for its own financial motives and flooded scholarly communication with a flurry of low quality and questionable research" [37].

I did not reply to the publisher's invitation and I advise even the most desperately aspiring medical writer to do the same. Don't say no (and thus confirm your e-mail address for them); just delete the message. Sad to say, there are some—just a few— less than honorable individuals in medical publishing, and the medical writer must always exercise due diligence with any offer, especially if it seems just a little too appealing. And maybe slightly off the mark.

I Have Received an Offer from a Well-Known, Prestigious Medical Publisher to Compile an Edited Reference Book in an Area in Which I Have Published Often. This Seems a Perfect Fit for My Abilities. How Should I Approach This Offer?

This offer is quite different from the one described just above, and it merits careful consideration, even if your eventual decision is to pass on the opportunity.

Over the past 40 years, I have edited some 15 multi-author medical reference books, 6 of them containing more than 1000 pages. I have coaxed and threatened authors. I have heard every tardiness excuse you can imagine—including one manuscript washed away in a flood. One author flagrantly lied to me for months, "My chapter is almost done; I'll have it to you next week." It never arrived. At manuscript submission time, another author exclaimed, "You weren't really serious about deadlines, were you?" I have suffered warring coauthors, and have had authors whose lives fell apart or even, unfortunately, died during manuscript preparation. I have done some very heavy editing on poorly written chapters, and not all authors were thrilled with my changes. Being the editor of a multi-author book is not for the faint of heart.

On the other hand, medicine needs courageous individuals willing to compile multi-author works. Every specialty needs a few of these. Today, with electronic manuscript preparation, submission, editing, proofreading, and even online revising when errors are found following publication, things are much easier than in the past. No more manuscripts "lost in the mail" or washed away in floods. And there are few things as thrilling as seeing your own multi-author work come together and be published. Now, if only authors could just get their contributions in on time.

If you decide to become a volume editor of a reference work, here are Dr. Taylor's ten rules to guide you to a timely, rewarding conclusion [38]:

- **Personal planning**: Organize your personal schedule as you plan the project. An edited book in not a steady effort. There are three very time-intensive phases; in between there are quiet times. The busy stages are (1) author recruitment, (2) manuscript editing, and (3) proofreading of book pages. These will not be good times to book a month-long ocean cruise.

- **Author selection**: Choose the author for each chapter with care. Match each author with a topic that he or she wants to "claim" in the literature. Even if you, the editor, are not well known, the prospective author will often agree to write the chapter, because that person knows that a refusal means you will offer the topic to someone else.
- **Recruiting authors**: Be firm in recruiting only authors committed to the project. An eager assistant professor may, in the end, be a better choice than the already over-committed senior faculty member. In the end, a late contributor responsible for a "must-have" chapter can delay the entire project. Early warning signs of potential tardiness in manuscript delivery are initial hesitation about the project, a long discussion about the many projects your possible author already has committed to do, and early attempts to negotiate a later deadline for manuscript submission. If you sense any of these "red flags," it might be best to go on to someone else.
- **Instructions to authors**: Provide crystal-clear instructions. Often the publisher has generic *Instructions to Authors*. You should consider creating your own supplementary instructions. For example: Do you want each chapter to begin with a quotation from Shakespeare or Osler? How many illustrations—if any—do you want in the chapter? How many reference citations are desired?
- **Page allocations**: Be very specific in your page allocations. If you tell the author you want, for example, a chapter of 20 manuscript pages, do you mean single-spaced or double-spaced pages? And does your page allocation include the Reference list at the end of the chapter, which can run to several manuscript pages?
- **Overwriting**: Beware of authors' tendency to write too many pages, even in spite of instructions any high school student could understand. It is hard to believe, but most authors tend to overwrite. Adding a few pages to the desired chapter length might not seem to be important, that is, until 50 or 80 or 100 authors all exceed page allocations, and the final book becomes a heavy tome. This has happened to me, as I described in Chap. 7.
- **What you do and don't want in the manuscripts**: Tell your authors your wishes about other things that may find their way into manuscripts: Do you want footnotes, or should all material be presented in the text? Would an Appendix to the chapter be acceptable? Will it be okay if authors thank their administrative assistants, spouses, or mentors?
- **Reminders**: Remind all authors monthly of the project. A real danger is that contributors forget about their chapters. After all, you gave the author a 6-month deadline, and so a natural tendency is to delay writing, focusing on more urgent issues such as teaching or seeing patients. Then, in a few months, the chapter you are counting on has become hazy in the author's memory. The way to avoid this is to send monthly reminders to all contributors. I tend to vary these: e-mails 1 month, postcards the next, letters the next, and so forth.
- **Following through**: After the edited work is published, be sure to thank your authors and confirm that each has received the promised copy of the book. If you promised authors a small fraction of the book's royalties (a practice which I do

not advise), be sure this pittance is received. Fractional royalties due contributors represent tiny payments; but there will be many of them, and the publisher's accounting department hates this practice. Nevertheless, if you made such a promise, be sure the publisher follows through.

- **Looking to the future**: Following publication, keep in touch with those who wrote for you, perhaps sending them copies of the book's glowing reviews. After all, you may want these authors to update their chapters in a few years or contribute to your next edited book.

What Are Some Classic Gaffes in the Medical Literature?

In Chap. 4, I described the Dizzy Awards, some slightly confusing contributions to the medical literature, and also the typographical, grammatical, and omission errors that somehow emerged in print. Here is another group of literary misadventures, some I consider to be more entertaining than simple obfuscation or misprints. These typically are wrong-headed misstatements and even ill-fated predictions. Wise medical writers keep in mind that what goes into print today may sound ridiculous when read back to you a few decades in the future.

Pierre Pachet was Professor of Physiology at Toulouse University in France and highly respected in his day. In 1872, however, he declared [39]:

> "Louis Pasteur's theory of germs is ridiculous fiction."

Benjamin Rush, sometimes called the "American Sydenham," was professor of chemistry at the Philadelphia Medical School, later to become the University of Pennsylvania Medical School. He wrote America's first chemistry book. Rush was an American patriot who signed the Declaration of Independence and served as Surgeon General of the Continental Army. But in 1796, he declared [40]:

> "I have formerly said there is but one fever in the world. Be not startled, Gentlemen, follow me and I will say there is but one disease in the world. The proximate cause of disease is irregular convulsive ... action in the [vascular] system affected."

JAMA has an engaging column titled "JAMA Revisited," transcribing verbatim articles published in the distant past. (I would enjoy the column even more if the original authors were identified more often.) My small criticism notwithstanding, I read it regularly and was amused by an article on bicycles, published in the August 15, 1896, issue of JAMA [41]:

> "The esthetics and morality of bicycling do not come within the professional ken of the physician. A costume and posture which make ninety women in a hundred absurd spectacles will not long be popular with the thousands and tens of thousands of that fair sex as today ... It is enough for us to declare that a woman, especially an adolescent girl, can not be suspended on the summit of a wedge without injury to the structures above, and the deformation of the pelvis; and that the bruising of the flesh, which some riders unwillingly admit, and the craving for stimulants after a fatiguing ride, ought to restrain the prevailing indiscriminate and intemperate use of the vehicle."

One of my favorite medical writers is Félix Martí-Ibáñez, medical writer and professor of the History of Medicine at the New York Medical College. Despite the erudition exhibited in his many works, including two quotations found in Chap. 9, in 1958 Martí-Ibáñez made the following prediction [42]:

"The profound change that is taking place in the natural history of infections warrants the prophecy that by the year 2000 the diseases caused by bacteria, protozoa, and perhaps viruses will be considered by the medical student as exotic curiosities of mere historical interest, as is the case today with tertiary syphilis, gout, and smallpox."

Baby and Child Care, the book by Benjamin Spock, influenced how many of us were raised. At the time of the early editions, Spock and the world of medicine were not yet aware of the sudden infant death syndrome (SIDS). Thus, in the 1958 edition of his book, Spock was simply being logical when he advised that infants not sleep while placed on their backs: "If (an infant) vomits, he is more likely to choke on the vomitus" [43].

In 1988, a molecular biology professor at University of California, Berkeley, is reported to have described the human immunodeficiency virus (HIV) as "a pussycat" [39].

How Often Are Medical Articles Retracted?

In Chap. 7, I described the fiasco of Andrew Wakefield's article, subsequently retracted, attempting to link childhood immunizations to developmental disorders. There have been many other retractions:

The *International Journal of Cardiology* has retracted a review article on pulsus paradoxus by Abu-Hilal et al. because "the authors have plagiarized part of a paper that had already appeared in *History of Medicine Online*" [44]. I followed the link to the 2006 victimized paper, a nice article by Woo et al. titled "Remarkable Physicians Associated With Pulsus Paradoxus, The Classic Sign—Richard Lower and Adolf Kussmaul" [45].

In July 2014, *Nature* issued a retraction of two papers it had published earlier in the year by Haruko Obokata et al. in Japan. The papers described an amazing break-through: creating embryonic-like stem cells from bodily cells by subjecting them to stress. Perhaps a little too amazing. The report of the retraction states, "The retrac-tions—agreed to by all of the co-authors—come at the end of a whirlwind 5 months during which various errors were spotted in the papers, attempts to replicate the experiments failed, the lead author was found guilty of misconduct, and the centre where she is employed was threatened with dismantlement" [46].

Steen et al. report a study of 2047 retracted scientific articles, which I find a very large number of discredited reports. They looked at the time to retraction from the date the article was published, finding that the more recently published articles are being retracted quicker, although the average retraction time for articles published after 2002 was still 23.82 months. (It seems *Nature*, as described above, acted with lightening speed.) Of interest was the finding that from 1993 to 2012, single-retraction authors wrote 63.1 % of retracted papers. In contrast, from 1972 to 1992, authors with a single retraction wrote 46.0 % of retracted papers, suggesting that during that earlier time there were more authors with multiple retractions. Steen et al. also note: "The first article retracted for plagiarism was published in 1979 and the first for duplicate publication in 1990, showing that articles are now retracted for reasons not cited in the past" [47].

Has There Ever Been a Fake Scientific Journal?

Yes, there have, in fact, been six fake medical journals. And that is just the ones we learned about. Here I am not writing about the open-access, "scan and spam," online predatory publications described in Chap. 5. By "fake scientific journals" I mean bogus, false, phony publications with a nefarious purpose, an intent even more egregious than convincing authors to pay for meaningless "publication" of their work. The goal for the fake journals was to introduce biased reports about pharmaceutical products into the literature. The hoax was perpetrated by an alliance of pharmaceutical companies and a cooperative journal publisher. Here is the story, and to be sure I am on sound legal ground, I am going to quote my sources liberally.

In 2009, Grant reported: "Scientific publishing giant Elsevier put out a total of six publications between 2000 and 2005 that were sponsored by unnamed pharmaceutical companies and looked like peer reviewed medical journals, but did not disclose sponsorship, the company has admitted" [48]. The author of the article goes on to describe one of the "journals": "The allegations involve the *Australasian Journal of Bone and Joint Medicine*, a publication paid for by pharmaceutical company Merck that amounted to a compendium of reprinted scientific articles and one-source reviews, most of which presented data favorable to Merck's products" [48].

In confirmation of the report by Grant, Huag, writing in the *New England Journal of Medicine* in 2013, told readers: "Until recently, 'international, scientific, peer-reviewed journal' has had a fairly specific meaning to the scientific community and to society at large: it has meant a journal that checks submitted papers for scientific quality, but also for relevance and interest to its readers, and also ensures that it contains new findings that may advance science. These features render a journal trustworthy and worthy of readers' time and money. Many observers were therefore understandably disturbed when the journal publisher Elsevier admitted in 2009 that it had published six 'fake journals' funded by pharmaceutical companies—in Elsevier's own words, 'sponsored article compilation publications … that were made to look like journals and lacked disclosure.' The company had intentionally exploited the word 'journal' to give the impression that these publications were honest and reliable" [49].

Will We Ever See Poems and Novels in Our Medical School Teaching and Clinical Practice?

I was prompted to consider this question by the words of nineteenth-century French physiologist Claude Bernard: "I feel convinced that there will come a day when physiologists, poets and philosophers will all speak the same language" [50] (see Fig. 10.5). Bernard, a pioneer of the scientific method and blinded experiments, promoted the concept of the *milieu intérieur*, what we now call homeostasis [52]. Before becoming a renowned scientist, however, he was an aspiring playwright, which may help explain his dream of universal interdisciplinary communication [53].

A century later, in his poem *Asphodel, That Greeny Flower*, William Carlos Williams wrote [54]: "It is difficult/to get the news from poems/yet men die miserably every day/for lack/of what is found there." What can we make of this? Williams, I believe, was not saying that a lack of what is found in poetry causes men to *die*, but rather that their deaths are sometimes unnecessarily miserable for want of the imagery, joy, and even the cadence of poems. And perhaps also, by inference, a paucity of philosophical reflection. In my opinion, he was writing about the quality of life at the time of dying, and how it can be enhanced by metaphor, simile, allusion, and nuance of language and thought.

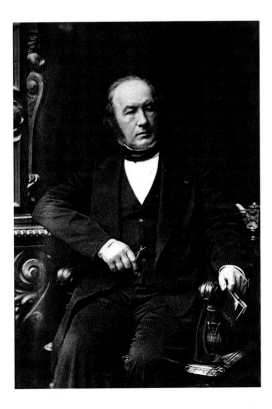

Fig. 10.5 French physiologist Claude Bernard, author of the book *Introduction to the Study of Experimental Medicine*, 1865 [51]

But, to return to Bernard, will we ever all speak the same language? I have written earlier in this book about the risks of creative prose in research reports. And isn't scientific language comprised largely of words that are polysyllabic, arcane, and derived from archaic Greek and Latin sources? These don't sound like the words of poets and philosophers. Or do they?

Poets speak of metre, caesura, iambic pentameter, alliteration, and (one of my favorite words) onomatopoeia. Philosophers speak of metaphysics and existentialism. Are these words any less inscrutable than words such as etiology, endothelial, musculoskeletal, prognosis, and other terms physicians use in their work and writings?

Ralph Waldo Emerson once called the poet "the true and only doctor," going on to explain about the poet: "He knows and tells; he is the only teller of news, for he was present and privy to the appearance which he describes. He is a beholder of ideas, and an utterer of the necessary and causal" [55]. But can the physician also have the heart of a poet? We seem to acknowledge this possibility by the inclusion of poetry and philosophy in many medical journals, and even on the program in some medical conferences.

Today many—perhaps most—medical schools offer courses that integrate medicine with literature and the humanities in general. In 1988, Calman et al. described one early course involving poems, plays, and books with both medical and non-medical themes [56]. In 2015, Stanford School of Medicine described their Arts, Humanities, and Medicine Program, offering "medical students, faculty, staff, and community members to explore the intersections between creative expression, humanities based critical inquiry, and value-driven social science with medicine and biosciences at Stanford" [57]. Now if we can only bring our diverse languages a little closer together.

What Is the Future for Medical Books, In Fact, Books of All Types?

Books will evolve. In the beginning they were hand-written, and later some were copied by scribes. Next came the printing press, with hand-set type. Production of books—actual paper books—became easier when everything "went digital," allowing many bound books now to be produced on demand; an order generates a printed book. Many books are currently read on *Kindle* and similar text readers. In fact, this book you are reading is available in print and also as an ebook. The future will bring new innovations. Maybe we will read books on our television sets, just as many of us now read the morning paper over breakfast. But whatever happens, the basic product will involve words that begin in the mind of an author and that, by some means, are organized into sentences, paragraphs, and completed works.

I Am Thinking About Becoming a Medical Writer. Are There Some Books and Websites That I Should Consult?

There are plenty of basic "how-to" books about medical writing, including one of mine (see below). Just search Google or Amazon. Among the many possibilities I have some favorites. Here I present seven diverse sources that may help someone considering medical writing as a serious endeavor. In the Appendix, there is also a list of books about language, sayings, writings, and the lore of medicine.

American Medical Writers Association Toolkit for New Medical Writers

The leading professional association of American medical writers, the American Medical Writers Association (AMWA), offers an informative website for aspiring medical writers. It is aimed at the person considering medical writing as a profession, rather than a health care professional contributing to the medical and scientific literature. But the topics discussed are, for the most part, important to all who consider themselves medical writers. These include types of medical writers, opportunities in medical writing, characteristics of successful medical writers, and resources available [58].

"A Writer's Toolkit," by Pories et al.

Pories and coauthors have given us a useful guide to writing in general, with a focus on down-to-earth, practical issues. They begin with a fundamental truism in writing: "The first step in any written scholarship is conceptualizing the scholarly project and establishing the importance of the topic." They go on to describe the literature search process, electronic resources, defining the scope of the project, establishing a timeline, selecting a target journal, and tips on how to submit your work for review [59].

"How to Become a Competent Medical Writer?" by Sharma

If I had been writing Sharma's title, I would not have included the question mark. But that minor criticism aside, I found this to be a comprehensive and readable overview of medical writing, which the author defines as "writing scientific documents of different types which include regulatory and research-related documents, disease or drug-related educational and promotional literature, publication articles like journal manuscripts and abstracts, content for healthcare websites, health-related magazines or news articles." In the article, he discusses types of medical writing, domain knowledge, steps in writing scientific documents, and available resources for medical writers [60].

"Been There, Done It, Got the T-shirt. The Life of a Medical Writer," by Woodrow

When I interview medical school applicants, I like to confirm that they understand the life that lies ahead. Not just the supposed glamour, but the long hours, hard work, and occasional disappointments. Ryan Woodrow, the author of this slide program, is a writer for a medical communications company who tells how he got into medical writing, the typical qualifications of medical writers, and how to find the job that is right for you. He ends the presentation with: "Each day I am writing or communicating about something different, and in doing so I am learning something new. Who needs more than that?" [61].

Recommendations for the Conduct, Reporting, Editing, and Publication of Scholarly Work in Medical Journals (ICMJE Recommendations)

The International Committee of Medical Journal Editors (ICMJE) "developed these recommendations to review best practice and ethical standards in the conduct and reporting of research and other material published in medical journals, and to help authors, editors, and others involved in peer review and biomedical publishing create and distribute accurate, clear, unbiased medical journal articles" [62]. The ICMJE recommendations are widely followed by journals, and any paper submitted that does not adhere to the advice given faces an uphill battle. Every medical writer aspiring to publication in a refereed scientific journal should be familiar with these recommendations.

Medical Writing: A Guide for Clinicians, Educators, and Researchers, 2nd Edition, by Taylor

Yes, this is my book. No list of recommended writing sources would be complete without listing a basic book in the field. Although written chiefly for an audience in academia, the book covers fundamental writing concepts such as idea development, article structure, technical issues in medical writing, and what's special about medical writing. There are also chapters on how to write a research protocol and how to write a grant proposal [38].

Aequanimitas and Other Addresses, by Osler

The book is a collection of addresses that Sir William Osler "delivered at sundry times and diverse places in the course of a busy life" [63]. The flagship address, for which the book is named, is "Aequanimitas," the word meaning "imperturbability," described as "coolness and presence of mind under all circumstances, calmness amid storm, clearness of judgment in moments of grave peril ...." It was the Valedictory Address to the University of Pennsylvania on May 1, 1889. Other addresses presented in the book include Osler's thoughts on "Teacher and Student," "Books and Men," and "The Hospital as a College" [63]. I include Osler's book, which saw its first edition printed more than a century ago, as an example of what medical writing can be.

What Innovation May Change the Paradigm of Medical Publishing?

Keep your eye on ReadCube, created by Labtiva, a software program that provides users an economically realistic way to view individual scientific papers, rather than subscribing to the entire journal or wait for an interlibrary loan. The Nature Publishing Group (publishers of *Nature*), Springer, Elsevier, and other leading publishing houses have announced participation [64]. The program, at least at this writing, allows a reader to view the article, but not to print, copy, or share the content—a model that Weintraub compares to the iTunes sales approach [65]. The ReadCube prototype can be a useful first step in combating the access-to-published-reports problem that scientists regularly encounter. Stay tuned.

If You Could Give Advice to Young Writers, What Would It Be?

1. Read every day, both to learn facts and also to study the writing style of successful authors.
2. Write every day, even if you think what you wrote today is not your best work. You can improve it tomorrow.
3. Marry someone or find a partner who likes your writing—both the product and also your doing it.
4. Edit your own work ruthlessly. Eliminate excess verbiage and strive for prose that is clean and clear.
5. Have fun writing. It can really be a great joy.
6. Don't worry about critical reviews; you know your work is good, even if it could be better.
7. Never give up. There is someone out there waiting to read your work.

References

1. Kahn RJ, et al. The Medical Repository—the first U.S. medical journal (1797–1824). N Engl J Med. 1997;337:1926.
2. Nejm18120101 Volume I Number I.jpg. This work is in the public domain in the United States, and those countries with a copyright term of life of the author plus 100 years or less. Available at: http://commons.wikimedia.org/wiki/File:Nejm18120101_Volume_I_Number_I.jpg.
3. About NEJM: past and present. Available at: http://en.wikipedia.org/wiki/Special:Search?search=&go=Go.
4. Highlights from the Bernard Becker Medical Library Collection. Available at: http://beckerexhibits.wustl.edu/rare/collections/periodicals.html.
5. Golden R. A history of William Osler's the principles and practice of medicine. Montreal: McGill University Osler Library studies in the history of medicine, No. 8; 2004.
6. Rare book consignments. Available at: http://www.rarebookconsign.com/OslerMedicine1892/.
7. John Elliotson, The principles and practice of medicine Wellcome L0028674.jpg. This file comes from Wellcome Images, a website operated by Wellcome Trust, a global charitable foundation based in the United Kingdom. This file is licensed under the Creative Commons Attribution 4.0 International license. Available at: http://commons.wikimedia.org/wiki/File:John_Elliotson,_The_principles_and_practice_of_medicine_Wellcome_L0028674.jpg.
8. Elliotson J. The principles and practice of medicine. 2nd ed. London: Butler; 1842.
9. Klems BA. Can I use a book title that's been used before? The Writers' Dig. Available at: http://www.writersdigest.com/online-editor/can-you-use-a-book-title-thats-been-used-before.
10. Fisher W. Medical journals are shifting from science to politics. Available at: http://www.kevinmd.com/blog/2013/01/medical-journals-shifting-science-politics.html.
11. Zuger A. A journal stands out in prestige and longevity. The New York Times/Science, 19 Mar 2012. Available at: http://www.nytimes.com/2012/03/20/science/200-years-of-the-new-england-journal-of-medicine.html?_r=0.
12. Dickson P. Authorisms: words wrought by writers. New York: Bloomsbury; 2014.
13. Menken HL. The American language: an inquiry into the development of English in the United States. 3rd ed. New York: Knopf; 1923.
14. Dickson P. Words from the White House. New York: Walker; 2013.
15. Hilton H. Sir Thomas Browne and the Oxford English dictionary. Oxford Dictionaries. Available at: http://blog.oxforddictionaries.com/2012/08/sir-thomas-browne/.
16. Online etymology dictionary. Available at: http://www.etymonline.com/index.php?term=staphylococcus.
17. Theodor Billroth NIH2.jpg. This image is in the public domain because its copyright has expired. Available at: http://commons.wikimedia.org/wiki/File:Theodor_Billroth_NIH2.jpg.
18. Mitchell SW. Phantom limbs. Lippincott's Mag. 1871;8:563–9.
19. Asimov I. Isaac Asimov's book of facts. New York: Bell; 1979. p. 503.
20. Keen H, et al. Urinary albumin excretion and diabetes mellitus. Lancet. 1964;2:1155.
21. Shem S. The house of God. New York: Dell Publishing; 1978.
22. Kaufman FR. Diabesity: the obesity-diabetes epidemic that threatens America—and what we must do to stop it. New York: Bantam; 2005.
23. Kurzweil R. The singularity is near. New York: Penguin; 2005.
24. Verghese A. Culture shock—patient as icon, icon as patient. N Engl J Med. 2008;359:2748.
25. Homogenic. In: Dictionary.com. Available at: http://dictionary.reference.com/browse/homogenic.
26. Lock SP. Journalology: are the quotes needed? CBE Views. 1989;12:57.
27. Biggs R, et al. Christmas disease: a condition previously mistaken for hemophilia. Br Med J. 1952;2:1378.
28. Todd J. The syndrome of Alice in Wonderland. Can Med Assoc J. 1955;73:701.
29. Alice par John Tenniel 11.png. This image is in the public domain because its copyright has expired. Available at: http://commons.wikimedia.org/wiki/File:Alice_par_John_Tenniel_11.png.

30. Rang M. The Ulysses syndrome. Can Med Assoc J. 1972;106:112.

31. Kuroki Y, et al. A new malformation syndrome of long palpebral fissures, large ears, depressed nasal tip, and skeletal abnormalities associated with postnatal dwarfism and mental retardation. J Pediatr. 1981;99:570.

32. Walsh B. MERS shows that the next pandemic is only a plane flight away. Time, 30 May 2014. Available at: http://time.com/87767/mers-shows-that-the-next-pandemic-is-only-a-plane-flight-away/.

33. Krause PJ, et al. Human Borrelia miyamotoi infection in the United States. N Engl J Med. 2013;368:291.

34. Stahl S. Mystery disease discovered locally, strikes mainly young women. CBS Philly, 7 Feb 2013. Available at: http://philadelphia.cbslocal.com/2013/02/07/health-mysterious-disease-discovered-locally-strikes-mainly-young-women/.

35. Martin M. Letter. Wall Street J. 7–8 June 2014, p. A12.

36. Personal Email message from publisher.

37. Wikipedia report. Available from: http://en.wikipedia.org/wiki/Bentham_Science_Publishers.

38. Taylor RB. Medical writing: a guide for clinicians, educators, and researchers. 2nd ed. New York: Springer; 2011.

39. Frater J. 15 extremely embarrassing science predictions. Available at: http://listverse.com/2010/12/22/15-extremely-embarrassing-science-predictions/.

40. King LS. The medical world of the eighteenth century. Chicago: University of Chicago Press; 1958.

41. JAMA revisited. Bicycling—pro and con. JAMA. 2014;312:99.

42. Martí-Ibáñez F. Men, molds and history. New York: MD Publications; 1958. p. 20.

43. Gilbert R, et al. Infant sleeping position and the sudden infant death syndrome: systematic review of observational studies and historical review of recommendations from 1940 to 2002. Int J Epidemiol. 2005;34:874.

44. Abu-Hilal MA, et al. RETRACTED: pulsus paradoxus; historical and clinical perspectives. Int J Cardiol. 2010;138:229.

45. Woo H et al. Remarkable physicians associated with pulsus paradoxus, the classic sign— Richard Lower and Adolf Kussmaul. Available at: http://priory.com/homol/pulsus.htm.

46. Cyranoski D. Papers on "stress-induced" stem cells are retracted. Nature. 2 July 2014. Available at: http://www.nature.com/news/papers-on-stress-induced-stem-cells-are-retracted-1.15501.

47. Steen RG, et al. Why has the number of scientific retractions increased? PLoS One. 2013;8(7):e68397. doi:10.1371/journal.pone.0068397.

48. Grant B. Elsevier published 6 fake journals. TheScientist. 7 May 2009. Available at: http://www.the-scientist.com/?articles.view/articleNo/27383/title/Elsevier-published-6-fake-journals/.

49. Haug C. The downside of open-access publishing. N Engl J Med. 2013;368:791.

50. Bernard C. Quoted in: Cousins N. The physician in literature. Philadelphia, PA: Saunders; 1982. Introduction page xxiii.

51. Claude Bernard.jpg. This image is in the public domain because its copyright has expired. Available at: http://en.wikipedia.org/wiki/Claude_Bernard.

52. Bernard C. Lectures on the phenomena common to animals and plants. Trans. Hoff HE et al. Springfield, IL: Charles C. Thomas; 1974.

53. Wilson DW. Claude Bernard. Pop Sci Mon. 1914;5:567.

54. Williams WC. Asphodel, that greeny flower and other love poems. New York: New Directions; 1994. First published in 1955.

55. Emerson RW. The poet. 1844. Available at: http://www.poetryfoundation.org/learning/essay/237846?page=2.

56. Calman KC, et al. Literature and medicine: a short course for medical students. Med Educ. 1988;22:265.

57. Medicine and the Muse: medical humanities and the arts. Stanford Center for Biomedical Ethics. Available at: http://bioethics.stanford.edu/arts/.

58. Toolkit for new medical writers. AMWA. Available at: http://www.amwa.org/toolkit_new_med_writers#Top1.

59. Pories S et al. A writer's toolkit. Available from: http://www.med.unc.edu/aoe/aoe-events/videos-and-materials-from-curricular-sessions/videos-and-materials-from-curricular-sessions-files/files-from-2012-2013/McMahon-A Writer-27s Toolkit Pories and Borus.pdf.
60. Sharma S. How to become a competent medical writer? Perspect Clin Res. 2010;1:33.
61. Woodrow R. Been there, done it, got the t-shirt. The life of a medical writer. Available at: http://www.slideshare.net/woodrowr/the-life-of-a-medical-writer-tips-for-people-considering-a-medical-writing-career.
62. Recommendations for the conduct, reporting, editing, and publication of scholarly work in medical journals. ICMJE. Available at: http://www.icmje.org/about-icmje/faqs/icmje-recommendations/.
63. Osler W. Aequanimitas and other addresses. 3rd ed. New York: Blakiston; 1932.
64. Lighten our darkness. The Economist, 6 Dec 2014, p. 92.
65. Weintraub K. A plan to open up science journals. The Boston Globe. 8 Oct 2012. Available at: http://www.bostonglobe.com/business/2012/10/07/start-readcube-program-uses-itunes-payment-model-for-access-scientific-articles/1UopCX1qfEE3uO2UEzuM7L/story.html.

Appendix A. Websites: The Medical Writer's Guide to the Internet

This is a list, corralled all in one place, of important websites described in the book:

Associations of Medical Writers

1. American Medical Writers Association. Available at http://www.amwa.org/about_us/.
2. European Medical Writers Association. Available at http://www.emwa.org/EMWA/About_Us/About_EMWA/EMWA/About_Us/About_EMWA.aspx?hkey=27ce6e80-c695-4062-8c9a-a37513e83c21.
3. Australasian Medical Writers Association. Available at http://www.wfsj.org/associations/page.php?id=262.

The Impact Factor

The Thompson Reuters Impact Factor. Web of Science. Available at http://wokinfo.com/essays/impact-factor/.

How to Prepare a Paper for a Scholarly Journal

Recommendations for the conduct, reporting, editing, and publication of scholarly work in medical journals. ICMJE. Available at http://www.icmje.org/about-icmje/faqs/icmje-recommendations/.

© Springer International Publishing Switzerland 2015
R.B. Taylor, *What Every Medical Writer Needs to Know*,
DOI 10.1007/978-3-319-20264-8

How to Calculate the Gunning Fog Index

http://gunning-fog-index.com/.

Open-Access Publication and Predatory Publishers

1. Beall J. Predatory publishers are corrupting open access. Nature. 2012;489:179.
2. Beale J. List of predatory publishers. Scholarly Open Access. Available at http://scholarlyoa.com/2014/01/02/list-of-predatory-publishers-2014/.
3. Bohannon J. Who's afraid of peer review? Science. 2013;342:60. Available at http://www.sciencemag.org/content/342/6154/60.full.

Duplicate Publication

Déjà vu: a database of highly similar citations. Virginia Bioinformatics Institute. Available at http://dejavu.vbi.vt.edu/dejavu/.

Plagiarism

CrossCheck Powered by iThenticate. Available at http://www.ithenticate.com/products/crosscheck/.

Conflict of Interest

Conflict of interest in biomedical research. The Hastings Center. Available at http://www.thehastingscenter.org/Publications/BriefingBook/Detail.aspx?id=2156.

Where to Find Figures That Are in the Public Domain

1. Wikimedia Commons. Available at http://commons.wikimedia.org/wiki/Main_Page.
2. Bing. Available at http://www.bing.com/images/.
3. Everystockphoto. Available at http://www.everystockphoto.com.

How to Start Your Own Medical Blog

How to start your medical blog: an introduction to the medblogosphere. RX Md Marketing Solutions. Available at http://rxmdmarketingsolutions.com/how-to-start-your-medical-blog-an-introduction-to-the-medblogosphere/.

Appendix B. Recommended Reading for the Serious Medical Writer

This is a list of books recommended for the reader interested in the legendary medical writers, the language of medicine, some of medicine's memorable sayings, and stories that may help you explain the historical context of current medical happenings. The books listed below are not "how-to-write" guides. Rather, they are books that will bring you an increased understanding of the legacy of medical knowledge that we enjoy, and thus may give greater depth to what you offer your reader. Each of these volumes has provided source material for at least one of my books.

Bean RB, Bean WB. Aphorisms by Sir William Osler. New York: Henry Schuman; 1950.

Bloomfield RL, Chandler ET. Pocket mnemonics for practitioners. Winston-Salem, NC: Harbinger Medical Press; 1983.

Bollett AJ. Plagues and poxes: the impact of human history on epidemic disease. New York: Demos; 2004.

Brallier JM. Medical wit and wisdom. Philadelphia: Running Press; 1994.

Breighton P, Breighton G. The man behind the syndrome. Heidelberg: Springer-Verlag; 1986.

Brody H. Stories of sickness. New Haven: Yale University Press; 1987.

Cartwright FF. Disease and history: the influence of disease in shaping the great events of history. New York: Crowell; 1972.

Dirckx JH. The language of medicine: its evolution, structure, and dynamics, 2nd edition. New York: Praeger; 1983.

Durham RH. Encyclopedia of medical syndromes. New York: Harper and Brothers; 1960.

Evans B, Evans C. A dictionary of contemporary American usage. New York: Random House; 1957.

Evans IH. Brewer's dictionary of phrase and fable. New York: Harper & Row; 1970.

Fabing HJ, Marr R, editors. Fischerisms, being a sheaf of sundry and diverse utterances culled from the lectures of Martin H. Fischer, professor of Physiology in the University of Cincinnati. Springfield, IL: Charles C. Thomas; 1937.

© Springer International Publishing Switzerland 2015
R.B. Taylor, *What Every Medical Writer Needs to Know*,
DOI 10.1007/978-3-319-20264-8

201

Firkin BG, Whitworth JA. Dictionary of medical eponyms. Park Ridge, NJ: Parthenon; 1987.

Fortuine R. The words of medicine: sources, meanings, and delights. Springfield, IL: Charles C. Thomas; 2001.

Garrison FH. History of medicine, 4th edition. Philadelphia: Saunders; 1929.

Gershen BJ. Word rounds. Glen Echo, MD: Flower Valley Press; 2001.

Haubrich WS. Medical meanings: a glossary of word origins. Philadelphia: American College of Physicians; 1997.

Holt AH. Phrase and word origins: a study of familiar expressions. New York: Dover; 1961.

Huth EJ, Murray TJ. Medicine in quotations: a view of health and disease through the ages. Philadelphia: American College of Physicians; 2006.

Johnson WM. The true physician: the modern doctor of the old school. New York: Macmillan; 1936.

Lindsay JA. Medical axioms, aphorisms, and clinical memoranda. London: H.K. Lewis Co.; 1923.

Magalini SI, Scrascia E. Dictionary of medical syndromes, 2nd edition. Philadelphia: Lippincott; 1981.

Maimonides M. Medical aphorisms: treatises 1–5, Bos G, editor. Provo, UT: Brigham Young University Press; 2004.

Major RH. Classic descriptions of disease, 3rd edition. Springfield, IL: Charles C. Thomas; 1945.

Maleska ET. A pleasure in words. New York: Fireside Books; 1981.

Manning PR, DeBakey L. Medicine: preserving the passion, 2nd edition. New York: Springer; 2004.

Martí-Ibáñez F. A prelude to medical history. New York: MD Publications; 1961.

Mayo CH, Mayo WJ. Aphorisms of Dr. Charles Horace Mayo and Dr. William James Mayo. Willius FA, editor. Rochester, MN: Mayo Foundation for Medical Education and Research; 1988.

McDonald P. Oxford dictionary of medical quotations. New York: Oxford University Press; 2004.

Meador CK. A little book of doctors' rules II. Philadelphia: Hanley & Belfus; 1999.

Meyers MA. Happy accidents. New York: Arcade Books; 2007.

Onions CT. The Oxford dictionary of English etymology. Oxford: Clarendon Press; 1979.

Osler W. Aequanimitas with other addresses. Philadelphia: Blakiston; 1906.

Pellegrino ED. Humanism and the physician. Knoxville, TN: University of Tennessee Press; 1979.

Pepper OHP. Medical etymology. Philadelphia: Saunders; 1949.

Reveno WS. Medical maxims. Springfield, IL: Charles C. Thomas; 1951.

Ross JJ. Shakespeare's tremor and Orwell's cough: the medical lives of great writers. New York: St. Martin's Press; 2012.

Sebastian A. The dictionary of the history of medicine. New York: Parthenon; 1999.

Shipley JT. Dictionary of word origins. New York: Philosophical Library; 1945.

Skinner HA. The origins of medical terms. Baltimore: Williams & Wilkins; 1949.

Silverman ME, Murray TJ, Bryan CS. The quotable Osler. Philadelphia: American College of Physicians; 2003.

Strauss MB. Familiar medical quotations. Boston: Little, Brown; 1968.

Taylor RB. White coat tales: medicine's heroes, heritage, heritage and misadventures. New York: Springer; 2008.

Taylor RB. On the shoulders of medicine's giants: what today's clinicians can learn from yesterday's wisdom. New York: Springer; 2015.

Train J. Remarkable words with astonishing origins. New York: Charles N. Potter; 1980.

Truss L. Eats, shoots & leaves: the zero tolerance approach to punctuation. New York: Gotham Books; 2003.

Weiss AB. Medical odysseys: the different and sometimes unexpected pathways to 20th century medical discoveries. New Brunswick, NJ: Rutgers University Press; 1991.

Acknowledgments

This is a book of reflections about medical writing, based on my personal experience in reading and putting words on my computer screen. But the wisdom, such as it is, behind my writing has been enhanced by those who have helped make me a better writer than I was when I penciled my first essays in Monongahela High School in Pennsylvania. Some of the names below are retired or residing in the celestial colony of writers and editors who spend eternity happily debating when a semicolon should be used or the merits of the occasional sentence in passive voice.

I owe a debt to my high school Latin teacher, Miss Martha E. Irwin, who did her best to nurture my interest in reading. I also thank my Bucknell University English professors Harry Garvin, John Wheatcroft, and Mildred Martin, who patiently corrected and graded my essays, yet who may remember me more as a basketball player than as a future author. My writing highlight was at Temple Medical School when, in response to an assignment to write a paper for a microbiology course, Professor Earle H. Spaulding allowed me to write on "A Philosophy for Microbiology," rather than a turgid treatise on bacteria or viruses. (The paper got an "A.")

I started writing books while engaged in a busy private family practice in upstate New York. My first book was *Feeling Alive After 65* (Arlington House Publishers, 1973), a health care guide written with my aging parents in mind. This was a trade book and several others followed, along with the obligatory television appearances, until medical editor Charles (Chuck) Visokay of Harper and Row Publishers recruited me to focus on books for medical professionals. These now number more than 30, including one of the two "big books" in my specialty, the edited reference book *Family Medicine: Principles and Practice,* with a seventh edition to be released soon.

Since I began writing and editing books for a health profession audience, most have been with my long-time publisher, Springer, and I thank the editors there who helped with this book, Katherine (Kate) Ghezzi, Margaret Moore, Janet Foltin, and Portia Wong, for their support.

© Springer International Publishing Switzerland 2015
R.B. Taylor, *What Every Medical Writer Needs to Know*,
DOI 10.1007/978-3-319-20264-8

I always recommend that a writer find a "critical reader," who will look over an article or book before it goes out for review. For me, that critical reader is my wife, Anita D. Taylor, MA Ed, author of the book *How to Choose a Medical Specialty*, currently in its fifth edition, plus a number of papers in peer-reviewed journals. Thank you, Anita, even when you advise me to remove what I think are my most brilliant sentences.

I am grateful for all the medical writers through the ages who have provided thought-provoking comments quoted in this book, and who have set high standards to which I continue to aspire.

Index

© Springer International Publishing Switzerland 2015
R.B. Taylor, *What Every Medical Writer Needs to Know*,
DOI 10.1007/978-3-319-20264-8

Printed in the United States
By Bookmasters